Out of the Blue

OUT
OF
THE
BLUE

A Memoir of Workplace Depression,
Recovery, Redemption and, Yes, Happiness

JAN WONG

Grateful acknowledgment is made for permission to reprint
excerpts from *Darkness Visible: A Memoir of Madness* by
William Styron, copyright © 1990 by Random House Inc.

Published in Canada by Jan Wong
Jacket design: Paul Hodgson
Text design: Paul Hodgson
Printed and bound in Canada
Published by Jan Wong. Visit her website at www.janwong.ca

To Gigi

Contents

Preface / 9

Part I: Fall
1. The Demon of Depression / 13
2. Tick Tock / 22
3. *L'Affaire Wong* / 33
4. A Threat Close to Home / 42
5. The Working Wounded / 53
6. Crack-Up / 63

Part II: Denial
7. The Geographic Cure / 71
8. Death by a Thousand Cuts / 77
9. Despair Beyond Despair / 88
10. Melancholia Through the Ages / 93
11. A Darker Shade of Blue / 102
12. The Music Cure / 115

Part III: Blue Print
13. A New Section Called "Life" / 126
14. Shrink-Fit / 136
15. Relapse / 141
16. Running in the Family / 151
17. Cipralex, Celexa, Effexor, Wellbutrin / 160
18. The Upside of Being Down / 169

Part IV: Healing
19. Fight or Flight? / 178
20. Smile, You're on Candid Camera / 184
21. Berries / 195
22. Flight, Again / 203
23. Year of the Rat / 210

Part V: Happiness
24. The Art of War / 218
25. Fired Up / 223
26. Hush Money / 228
27. Eat Bread. Butter, Too / 236
28. Roses / 243

Afterword / 252
Acknowledgments / 255
Selected Bibliography / 258

Preface

Out of the Blue is the story of my personal journey into and out of depression. The particular events that led to losing my job comprise the narrative thread, but the way I was treated is probably no different from the way many companies treat employees with a mental illness. In this book I have tried my utmost to be objective, to let the facts speak for themselves. Every scene, quotation and incident is based on documents, eyewitness accounts, interviews or my direct experience.

My goal is to bring you, the reader, into a depressive's emotional world. Some may dispute my interpretation of events. And, indeed, as I have written in this book, I know that a person's perception of reality becomes skewed during a major depressive episode. When I was depressed, I discovered that I was alternately hypersensitive and hyposensitive. I felt some things acutely, perhaps too acutely. At other times I misread cues. I acknowledge those occasions when I might have misinterpreted words and gestures, or where my emotional response to a situation was colored by depressive symptoms. What I present here is the most accurate narrative I could assemble based on the evidence.

There is no universal story of depression. That is why it's so hard to diagnose. It's why so many—friends, family and employers—are skeptical and pass judgment. Depression is a complicated illness. You may read what happened to me and think, *Hey! That's not what it's like.* But it runs the gamut from paralysis to high-functioning behavior, with many layers in between. Some people stay up all night to justify staying in bed all day. Others seem normal: they go to work, they socialize, they run errands. And then one day, they go home quietly and kill themselves. Wade Belak, an enforcer in the National Hockey League for ten seasons, lived an enviable life with a beautiful young family and a new gig as a host on an all-sports FM station in Nashville. He was in the midst of taping *Battle of the Blades*, a hit Canadian television show that pairs hockey players with figure skaters in an ice-dancing competition. On what would turn out to be the last night of his life, Belak went out to a bar with a friend. By all accounts he appeared in good spirits. Less than twelve hours later, when he failed to show up for a radio interview, staff at the Toronto condo where he was staying checked on him. They found he had hanged himself in his room.

"He was such a bright light," his former coach with the Toronto Maple Leafs, Pat Quinn, later told the *Toronto Star*. "He had a smile on his face every day."

I smiled, too, even when I despaired, although perhaps not every day. This book is not only about that descent into despair. It is also the story of my recovery. I am healthy now, and very productive. I want to tell you that there is day after night, and hope on the other side.

PART I

FALL

CHAPTER 1

The Demon of Depression

This letter is to let you know that I will be going soon to Toronto to kill you .... It will make me feel good to shoot at you a bullet right through your skull ...
p.s. I know where you live.

That's all I managed to read before I averted my eyes and called the police.

Four days later, I was still scared. On a quiet Sunday evening in October, as I pulled into my driveway in Toronto, I glanced at the rear-view mirror. A pickup truck, its headlights on, was parked across the street in the empty lot of the school—my children's school. My heart began to pound.

The killer has found my house.

Shaking, I pressed the remote control on the visor. The heavy blue garage door rumbled open. I drove in. I checked my rear-view mirror again, but the pickup truck hadn't moved. Its lights were still on.

To see better when he aims.

Inside the garage, sitting in my minivan, I assessed my options. A bullet would splinter the wooden garage door, shatter the van windows, smash into my skull. The brick walls of my house were thicker. I would take a chance and make a run for it. Carrying a purse, fumbling for a house key, would slow me down. I left my purse in the van. I swung open the van door, leapt out and dashed across the driveway, vaulting two steps to my front door.

Hurry! Please hurry, I prayed as I stabbed the small illuminated doorbell.

I had phoned ahead to say I'd be home in half an hour. Normally I don't do that, but the death threat had changed everything. I couldn't remember whether my husband or one of the boys had answered the phone. Whoever it was had merely grunted when I said I was on my way. I didn't say—didn't want to say out loud—*someone is trying to kill me.* I knew my family would understand I meant for them to wait at the door.

Where were they? I pressed my nose to the sidelight. I stabbed the doorbell again, so hard the tip of my finger turned white. Still no one came. Leaving my purse—and house key—in the van was a fatal error. Now if I ran back, my killer could shoot me on the way. What if he cornered me in the garage?

Perhaps I would not get shot if I didn't look back? *Don't turn around.* That's what the bad guys always say in the movies. And then a ridiculously long conversation ensues and the victim escapes. This could work for me: I would not turn around and I would escape. Except that the killer hadn't agreed to any deal.

It will make me feel good to shoot at you a bullet right through your skull.... *p.s. I know where you live.*

On a subconscious level, even as I was trying not to get killed, I couldn't help parsing the sentence. My inner editor itched to cross out the words, "at you." The journalist in me made a mental note: English is not his native tongue. Perhaps he is a French speaker. When translated literally, "to shoot a bullet at you" becomes perfectly acceptable French: *tirer une balle sur toi.* (I assumed the killer was male: we journalists know that men issue death threats, not women.)

This was, however, no time for fixing grammar. I leaned on the doorbell with all my strength. In the silence of the autumn evening, I could hear the long, strident ring, as shrill as a panic button in an elevator.

Still no one came.

I began screaming. I banged on the door, bruising my knuckles. The blue-painted steel, insulated against Canadian winters, muffled the sound of my pounding. I was crying now, tears of pure terror. Did no one care if I died? I became convinced the killer was now standing right behind me. I still believed if I didn't turn around, I had a chance. Time passed. It might have been eight seconds or eight minutes. I had no idea.

Through the sidelight, I saw my husband bounding down the stairs. He seemed confused and alarmed as he unlocked the door. My fear turned to rage.

"Why didn't you open the door?" I screamed.

Norman looked astonished, but he had the presence of mind to spread the blame. "We didn't hear you."

I stormed past him. Our two teenage boys, Ben and Sam, were standing together at the top of the stairs. Both looked bewildered.

"Why didn't you open the door?" I screamed. I was trembling, my face wet with tears. The words "pickup truck," "killer" and many others tumbled incoherently from my mouth.

"Sorry," said Ben, sixteen years old, looking stricken. "We didn't hear the bell." He had been watching a movie on his laptop, headphones on, door closed. Sam, thirteen years old, had been in the shower. Norman had been in his office handling household bills, while listening to Bach's Goldberg Variations on his computer.

It was a normal Sunday evening, but I was beyond comprehending their explanations.

"Why didn't you open the door?" I screamed again and burst into fresh tears.

Not one of them dared ask the reasonable question: why didn't you use your key? Instead, Sam, still damp from the shower, wrapped me in a bear hug. He held me tightly until I finally stopped shaking.

I know, of course, how to use a key. I live in one of the safest communities on the planet. Except for one domestic homicide a few years back, there hasn't been a murder in my neighborhood in, well, no one can remember how long, not even my friend Edward J. Carter, and he was elected city councilor in 1949 and has the most remarkable memory of anyone I know. I don't consider myself the hysterical type. As they say in the journalism business, I am a tough cookie. Scary situations are part of my job. I know that if I don't take risks, I won't get stories. I covered the 1989 massacre at Tiananmen Square. I tracked Canada's first SARS victims (and ended up in quarantine myself).

Some of my past articles had sparked death threats. When this happened, I would scan the rooftop parking lot as I left the office. But I always kept my equilibrium. One caller, for reasons I never understood, filled my voice mail at work with threatening messages. I ignored them until one day he announced, "I'm going to roast you alive." That seemed a tad graphic so I reported his name and phone number—yes, I knew who he was—to my newspaper's security chief, who phoned the man back and then reported the threat to the police. The calls stopped. The incident was no big deal. I never forgot the barbecuing bit, but it didn't send me into a tailspin either. I moved on.

This time something inside me had changed. In recent days I had received hundreds of pieces of hate email. Then an anonymous package arrived at the office that shocked and disturbed me. The *coup de grâce* was the bullet-right-through-your-skull threat.

The old me would have spotted the fallacy instantly: "p.s. I know where you live." If the killer knew that, why send the threat to my office?

The old me would have spotted another fallacy. If he was so intent on killing me, why warn me?

My brain had stopped functioning. If the old me had spotted a suspicious vehicle, I would have driven straight to the closest police station, calling the cops en route. Had I been trapped inside my garage, the old me would have shut the garage door and called 911 from inside. At the very least, the old me would never have jumped out of the van without my keys. Indeed, I would have spiked them between my fingers as improvised brass knuckles, the way I'd once been taught in a self-defense class at university. But for reasons I am only now beginning to understand, I was not the old me. I was so scared I couldn't get into my house without help.

Out of the blue, everything had changed. My life had unraveled.

Here's the short version: I wrote a feature story that sparked a political backlash, my employers failed to support me and later silenced me, and after I became clinically depressed, they fired me.

There. I summed up the story in one sentence. I must be getting better.

For a scarily long time, I was a writer who couldn't write. And if I couldn't write, who was I? When I was sick, my memory frayed and then disintegrated. I would start to say something, and then stop. I couldn't finish my sentence because I had no idea what I had just been talking about. I lost more than the ability to have a conversation. I left my credit card with the cashier in shops. I misplaced my car keys. I lost my mind.

Friends tried to comfort me by telling me how they had mislaid their reading glasses. It was no comfort. Normal for me was keeping absolute control of my life. In thirty years, I had never been sick for more than a day at a time. But now as I fell apart, my family doctor, and then a psychiatrist, and then another psychiatrist, diagnosed me with severe depression. The doctors called it "M.D.E." It stood for "major depressive episode."

The panic attack outside my home was just the beginning. Depression robbed me of my ability to think coherently. I would spend an entire day composing one short email. My tears, forgetfulness and hysterical rages bewildered my family and friends. No one understood what clinical depression meant. Even I didn't understand. It took me eight months to accept the doctors' diagnosis and start treatment. As I fell into a deep melancholy and lost the capacity to function in a newsroom, my employer suspected me of malingering and then its insurer accused me of the same thing. This affected me deeply. It seemed to call into question my very integrity—the only capital any reporter has—and intensified and prolonged my depression.

Yet something at my core remained a journalist. Even when I was sick and staying at home, I filed away ticket stubs, maps and receipts. I hoped these bits of paper would provide a record of what I did and where I went. And although I couldn't write stories, I never stopped observing and listening. Whenever I heard a good quote or noticed a telling detail, a light bulb would still switch on in my befuddled brain. As I got better, I began jotting things down, fragments of conversations, the time and date when something significant happened, how I was feeling from one day to another. As Virginia Woolf wrote in *The Years*, the last novel published in her lifetime, "Take notes, and the pain goes away."

After many months at home, it occurred to me that writing *about* my depression might help me to claw my way *out* of depression. My literary agent did not think it advisable. "It will reopen the wounds," he said. By then I had been seeing a psychiatrist weekly for more than a year. I asked for his opinion. "Your wounds aren't closed," my doctor said, neither encouraging nor discouraging me.

In the end, I felt I had no choice. If I did not vanquish depression by writing about it, I feared I would never write again. I sat down at my computer and managed three sentences, the first writing I had managed in eight months:

I am an outspoken reporter who is forbidden to speak out and can no longer write. I don't live in Burma or North Korea. I live in Canada, a tolerant, mild-mannered, accommodating, apathetic and slightly apologetic democracy.

Hmm. A bit overblown, but the idea was there, and so was a hint of a sense of humor. Like the first steps of a stroke victim, the sentences were unsteady, but at least I seemed to be moving forward.

Many people assume there is something powerfully therapeutic in writing about depression. I haven't found it so, not while I was writing, anyway. In his 1947 essay entitled, "Why I Write," George Orwell noted, "Writing a book is a horrible, exhausting struggle, like a long bout of some painful illness. One would never undertake such a thing if one were not driven on by some demon whom one can neither resist nor understand." Writing about the demon of depression forced me to relive my illness, moment by moment. On some days, I would lapse into the condition I experienced at the nadir of my depression—quick to anger, close to tears, unable to sleep. It was very hard on my family. I felt the therapeutic effect eventually when the book was done. Completing it felt liberating, peaceful even. I could finally forget about it, knowing that, if I ever needed to remember what had happened, the record was there. In her research, Shelley H. Carson, a psychology professor at Harvard University, has found that writers and artists are spurred to create *after* their recovery from depression, not during the illness itself.

My previous experience of writing books had been smooth and pleasurable, a chance to let the creative juices flow, to take enough space to convey the colors, textures and characters I had had to cut from my newspaper stories. This time the writing process was ineffably difficult. I labored over the first painful draft for months. And after all that effort, the manuscript was meandering, incoherent, vindictive and obsessive. It could not even be edited. I filed it away as an historical relic and never looked at it again. My subsequent attempts took many more months. I wrote multiple drafts and endured (or my editor endured) several major rewrites.

In this book, I chart my personal journey into and out of depression. How does the disease manifest itself? How does it wreak havoc on one's life? How is it different from ordinary sadness? How does one cope with the loss of a job that has been central to one's identity? I am not a psychologist, psychiatrist or social worker. I am a writer. I can only document what happened to me: I loved my work. It defined me. It was my life. I lost my job but I didn't lose my life. I recovered and I gained a new identity.

Whenever I can, I delve into current research and explore the larger issues. I discuss what is common to humanity and even to baboons, for there is compelling evidence that animals suffer from stress and depression, too. I hope that by illuminating the dark corners of this disease, I can help others. At the very least, by going public myself, I know I will erase a bit of the terrible stigma attached to this illness.

Depression is not a new affliction. It has plagued humanity since the beginning of recorded history, and more. It crosses all cultures. It transcends economic and geographic boundaries. It affects people in the poorest nations and those in the richest. It is frightening, serious, life threatening, family shattering and soul destroying. Yet those who have it are often regarded with suspicion, in part because depression doesn't look or feel like a *real* disease, in part because ignorance breeds fear. An inability to interact with the world doesn't seem as serious or debilitating as, for example, cancer, despite high mortality rates for both conditions. Indeed, some people still view depression as an affliction of the leisure class. There is a sense that visiting a psychiatrist is self-indulgent, more like visiting a manicurist than an oncologist. If that is the perception, it is only because the elite are better equipped to talk about and address the illness. A cashier, a plumber and a journalist may all suffer from depression, but the latter is most likely to write about it.

In fact, the poor suffer from the highest rates of depression because poverty is, well, inherently depressing. Poverty, of course, is relative. And in the West, and many parts of the East, as the rich get richer and the poor get poorer, rates of depression are on the rise. In the century preceding the 1970s, the average American male worker was generally better off than his father. Then everything changed. By the 1980s, wages became stagnant in real terms, even as corporate profits swelled. To compensate for lower real wages, fathers worked longer hours. Then mothers joined the workforce and did the same. Two-income families assumed unprecedented debt. By the 1980s, college students in the United States told researchers their number one goal was no longer "developing a meaningful philosophy of life," as it had been ever since the Great Depression. Instead, their top goal became "being very well off financially" and this remains the case today.

All this striving and insecurity take an enormous toll.

Depression is astonishingly, breathtakingly pervasive. It directly or indirectly affects the lives of virtually everyone in the world. It is, writes University of Pennsylvania psychologist Martin Seligman, "the common cold of psychopathology." Depression is now second only to heart disease as the leading cause of disability. The World Health Organization forecasts that one in ten of the world's six billion people will suffer from a major depressive episode at some point in their life. In the United States, half of all Americans will experience some symptoms of depression. In Canada, one in every five or six people will experience clinical depression. In China, where until recently the word was rarely mentioned, nearly 15 percent of middle school students have reported suffering from depression, according to a survey conducted by the Nanjing Center for Disease Prevention and Control.

Before I got sick myself, I had no clue how widespread depression is. I knew of only two friends who were seeing a psychiatrist, one for schizophrenia, the other one for marital and career problems. I didn't know anyone who suffered from clinical depression. Let me rephrase that. I didn't *know* that I knew anyone who had suffered from depression. No one had ever revealed to me that they had been depressed, except maybe my mother, and she had told me only in passing, when I was young and thoughtless and too startled to ask for details. But when I became depressed and refused to cover up my condition, people suddenly began to confide in me. They described their own experiences or told me about sufferers in their families. It was as if I had discovered the secret handshake to an underground society.

"For a lot of people, for a very long time, depression was a hidden and masked illness because it's a *mental* illness," says Patricia Kirby, a retired psychotherapist in Toronto.

Like so many sufferers, I was affected by the stigma. The words "mental illness" scared me. I thought depression meant you were nuts. I thought it only afflicted the weak. I was strong, so it could never happen to me, right?

Forgive me. My ignorance seems improbable for a baby boomer. Perhaps my naiveté was the result of living in China for most of the 1970s, a watershed decade in Western culture. In 1972, fascinated by Mao's Cultural Revolution, I moved from my hometown of Montreal to Beijing to see it for myself—and stayed for most of the next eight years. The long sojourn abroad meant that I missed large pieces of my generation's collective cultural awakening. I cannot, for instance, name a single hit song by ABBA, Queen, Pink Floyd or AC/DC because I wasn't around at the height of their popularity. Lacking a rock-band vibe is not a big deal. More problematically, I missed the 1970s revolution in cognitive psychology and the birth of behavioral medicine and health psychology. That is why, before my own experience with depression, I knew nothing about its causes or symptoms.

Like most journalists, I am curious. But when I was depressed, I did not want to read about depression. My curiosity, like the rest of me, was half-dead. I avoided research for another reason, too. I feared that if I learned that depressed people suffered from insomnia, for instance, I would become an insomniac myself. When I decided to write this book, however, I began to read voraciously. I learned there are two main kinds of depression. One is a milder form that occurs gradually and sometimes becomes chronic. The other is a severe, sudden breakdown. That was the kind I had.

In *The Noonday Demon: An Atlas of Depression*, Andrew Solomon compares the soul to an iron structure and severe depression to rust, causing "the startling collapse of a whole structure." I experienced a total structural collapse. But here's the surprising and scary aspect of depression: it doesn't afflict only the weak. The strong are just as vulnerable. In fact, susceptibility to depression has nothing to do with strength or weakness. And yet, many people persist in equating weakness with vulnerability, and strength with invulnerability. Certainly, that confused many around me because before I fell sick, no one would have described me as weak.

What happened to me is proof that depression can strike no matter how strong, able and tough-minded someone is. I was hardy. I thrived on deadline pressure. I loved working at my newspaper and had been there for nearly twenty years. I happily thought of myself as a feminist workaholic. I rationalized away the long hours I spent building my career by seeing the dual roles of mother and journalist as complementary, not conflicting. Okay, so I wasn't always there to play Lego with my children. But by being focused, conscientious and hardworking, I could be a role model for them. I could show them the rewards of a fulfilling career.

I fancied myself a truth-teller, a crusader even. Each success, each front-page byline produced a pleasurable jolt. Practicing journalism was like being on drugs. To maintain that adrenalin high, I worked long hours, put my job first and scorned those who didn't. I lapped up the recognition, such as it was. People stopped me to say hello on the subway or in the lineup for the ladies' room at my local multiplex. It wasn't much, but I felt flattered and it validated my identity.

Then around noon on a gray Wednesday in September, my life changed. A twenty-five-year-old man stormed into Dawson College in Montreal and shot twenty people. It was a horrendous, shocking crime. The next day, my editors put me on the story. I assumed it would be just another assignment in my newspaper career. In fact, for my career and my mental health, it was the beginning of the end.

CHAPTER 2

Tick Tock

The night before the last day of his life, Kimveer Gill stayed up late chatting on-line and listening to heavy metal music. He was twenty-five, a hollow-eyed young man of East Indian descent who shaved his thick, dark hair at the sides and lived in his parents' basement in suburban Montreal. Nine months earlier in an on-line journal, he had declared that the day he planned to seek revenge would be gray.

"A light drizzle will be starting up," he had written.

That next morning, it rained. Gill donned black jeans, combat boots and a long, black *Matrix*-style trench coat that emphasized his slim, six-foot-one build. Just before noon, he loaded three guns and a package of ammunition into the trunk of his black Pontiac sports car. He then drove twenty minutes downtown to Dawson College, a provincially funded university-preparatory institution known as a CEGEP, the French acronym for *Collège d'enseignement général et professionnel* (College of General and Vocational Education).

The CEGEP, a uniquely Québécois school, provides two-year programs, free of charge, to high-school graduates before they enter university. Gill himself had attended CEGEP—not Dawson—for one semester and had dropped out. Now he was unemployed. Records later showed that he had acquired his armory legally: a Glock .45-calibre handgun, a Chinese-made Norinco HP9-1 short-barreled shotgun and a Beretta Cx4 Storm semi-automatic carbine. The Beretta, his favorite, could fire ten rounds without having to be reloaded.

In 2006, Dawson, one of only five English-language CEGEPs, had about ten thousand students, mostly aged seventeen and eighteen. Located in Westmount, Montreal's wealthiest and most exclusive enclave, the college occupies a sprawling, century-old, yellow-brick building once owned by the Grey Nuns of Montreal. Gill parked on Wood Avenue, a narrow tree-lined residential street on the western edge of the campus. He opened his trunk and unloaded his arsenal. He stashed the ammunition and all the guns except the Beretta in a large black canvas bag. Gripping the semi-automatic carbine in one hand, he slammed the trunk shut and slung the bag over his shoulder.

A group of teenage boys stood halfway down the block, idly watching. Gill stared at them for a moment. Then he raised the Beretta to his shoulder, and took aim through the scope. The boys saw him, but didn't move. One of them later said he thought the gun was a toy.

Gill lowered his gun. He strode along the sidewalk on de Maisonneuve Boulevard, the one-way street bordering the south edge of the campus. His route took him past a fenced area of picnic tables and playground dinosaurs belonging to Dawson's daycare center. The grounds were deserted. Perhaps the rain had kept the toddlers inside. A few seconds later, he reached the main entrance of the college. There he shot at point-blank range two students who were smoking outside. It was 12:41 P.M. Gill swung open the heavy glass doors and entered the atrium, which was teeming with students on their lunch break. He fired his Beretta again, this time into the crowd. Then he turned right and entered the busy cafeteria, where he continued shooting. One of his victims was an eighteen-year-old commerce student named Anastasia De Sousa. As she lay on the floor bleeding, one of her classmates, a young man named James Santos, tried to drag her behind a serving counter.

"Is she still alive?" Gill asked. "Today is the day she's going to die."

He shot her eight more times.

My editors knew Montreal was my hometown. Within moments of the shooting, they also knew I had an inside source. My sister, Gigi, teaches business at Dawson College. Luckily, she didn't have classes that day and was safely at home. She only learned a gunman was inside the building when a colleague called her in hysterics. Pina Salvaggio was sobbing, nearly incoherently, because she hadn't been able to reach her son, a Dawson student, who was somewhere in the building. She had barricaded herself inside the office she shared with my sister, along with several terrified students who had ducked in from the hall. They were all cowering inside, convinced the killer was right outside the door because the atrium's open plan pushed the *rat-tat-tat* sound straight up.

Gigi told Pina to stay put while she called 911. Then my sister called me. "I just want you to know I'm at home and I'm okay."

"That's nice," I said. I had just returned to my desk after having lunch with a friend.

"Haven't you heard?" my sister asked, impatiently.

I listened in shock.

"Are you okay?"

"I'm at home," she repeated. "I don't have classes on Wednesday."

When stories break, journalists scramble. I knew the national desk would be frantic for sources, details, firsthand information. I urged my sister to talk to the national news desk. Reluctantly she agreed, which is how my editors discovered I had an inside source.

The next day, when a senior editor told me to get on a plane to Montreal, I felt the familiar adrenalin rush. When everyone else is running from danger, reporters rush toward it. As I dashed to the airport, my only regret was that I was already one day behind the competition.

I loved seeing things firsthand.

The summer I was nineteen, I traveled alone to China and surprised everyone, including myself, by becoming the first Canadian to study there during the Cultural Revolution. I stayed a year, returned home to finish my history degree at McGill University and then went right back to China for more studies at Peking University. In 1979, my Mandarin and my familiarity with China got me a job as a news assistant at *The New York Times*' newly opened Beijing bureau.

I discovered I adored journalism. A year later, impatient for my own byline, I quit the *Times*, moved to New York City and earned a master's degree from Columbia University's School of Journalism. From there, I landed staff-reporter jobs at the Montreal *Gazette*, *The Boston Globe* and *The Wall Street Journal*. My goal was to return to China as a foreign correspondent. Unfortunately, neither of the first two newspapers could afford an office in Beijing. And soon after I joined *The Wall Street Journal*, the editors in New York decided—this is true—that there was insufficient news coming out of China and shut down the bureau. That's how I ended up applying for a job at *The Globe and Mail* in Toronto. I knew it had a Beijing bureau. In fact, it had maintained an outpost in the Chinese capital ever since 1959. The editors assured me they had no plans to close the office. So in 1988, I joined the *Globe* and moved to Toronto. Less than a year later, the editors appointed me the newspaper's thirteenth Beijing bureau chief.

I loved working as a reporter. My job provided freedom, fun and a generous expense account. One day I would be in Florida investigating a cult called the Raelians who believed in human cloning. Another day, I'd be in Ulan Bator covering Mongolia's first elections. I enjoyed an independence that was virtually extinct among the salaried classes. I was free to voice my opinions *and* I got paid to express them. I had moderate influence, too. I could save the little guy and deep-six the bad guy. On a good day, I could make readers either laugh out loud or shed a tear. I loved racing the clock, squeezing out one more phone call, one last rewrite before the deadline.

Like any high-pressure, high-reward job, journalism was addictive. When my colleagues and I hadn't had a story in the paper for a while, we would talk about "severe byline deprivation." The withdrawal symptoms were almost physical, and the effect was to drive us to work long hours in the hopes that our next story would make the front page. I never tired of covering the news, but my obsession with work was a vice masquerading as a virtue.

By the time the Dawson story broke in 2006, I had spent nearly thirty years in the business. I measured my life by my work. Published corrections are a professional humiliation: I can remember every single one in my career, but at some point I realized I couldn't recall when my firstborn son began to walk. Was I off covering a story in Sichuan province at the time? I am ashamed to report that I measured death by my work, too. In the midst of my depression, on the anniversary of my mother's passing, I couldn't remember the year she had died and determined it was the fourth anniversary only by recalling a story I had written at the time and checking the date of its publication.

I never realized how obsessed I was. To me journalism was the best job I ever had. In fact, it was the only job I ever had.

I had twenty-four hours to churn out a three-thousand-word story. In the taxi on my way to the airport, I called the national editor to discuss the assignment. "Do you want a tick-tock?" I asked, meaning a blow-by-blow re-creation. "Or do you want a *New Yorker*-style magazine piece with analysis?"

"We want both," the national editor said. "We definitely want analysis."

I knew Dawson College would be sealed off as a crime scene. But I also knew I could rely on my sister. With her help, I could tell readers the color of the cafeteria walls, map the killer's path through the building, contact others who worked there. Through her, I would also have some idea what the administration was telling students and teachers.

Gigi is the youngest of four kids. My brother, Earl, is the oldest; I'm second; and my brother, Ernie, is the third. Because there is a five-year gap between us, Gigi and I never played together as kids. But as sisters we have always been a team. She remembers me as her schoolyard protector against a bully at Sir Arthur Currie Elementary School. I remember she slipped me a muffin and apple when I was about ten and Mom punished me for some misdemeanor by sending me to bed without supper.

My sister and I have a special bond. I was working at my first newspaper, the Montreal *Gazette*, when she took the grueling exams at McGill University to become a chartered accountant. Back then the failure rate was a brutal 50 percent and Gigi couldn't face going in person to check the results when they were posted. Instead, she arranged for a classmate to call at 9 A.M. the day the marks came out—but only if the news was good.

The night before, Gigi bunked over at my downtown apartment. We slept fitfully. At 9 A.M., we were wide awake, but too afraid to get out of bed. As the minutes ticked by, we waited. And waited. Twelve of the longest minutes passed, and then the phone rang. Her friend had been so thrilled by her own good news that she had called her family first.

We were a tag-team then and later. When Gigi was going through her divorce, I flew to Montreal for the court date and helped stare down her ex. I backed her that day when she decided to accept absurdly low child support in exchange for full custody, her chief concern. But when the law on minimum child support subsequently changed, I informed my sister, who went back to court and effortlessly had her monthly allotment increased.

Although I don't think we look alike, everyone instantly sees that we are sisters. We are the same height—five feet, three inches—and we both wear glasses, but there the resemblance ends. Her hair has a silken sheen; mine is dull and flyaway. I envy her size 7-1/2B feet; mine are 8EE, which means that nothing sleek and sexy ever fits. Gigi likes to read mysteries and watch "Judge Judy" on television. I prefer non-fiction and foreign films. I used to think I was shrewd at sizing people up, but I now know she is shrewder. She can spot a phony instantly.

As a chartered accountant, she is good at math, money and taxes. She can parallel park. And, having taken a two-year professional carpentry course, she can even build a staircase. All I can do is write. Yet Gigi admires *me*. Before my crisis, she described me as the successful one in the family. Over the years, she has always been there for me—cheerleader, helper, key advisor, even on occasion a chauffeur, interior designer and beauty consultant. When I was sent to Montreal to cover the ice storm of the century, I was too chicken to get behind the wheel, so Gigi drove me along unplowed roads under cracking tree branches through the blacked-out city. When I renovated my kitchen, she suggested installing two dishwashers so I would never waste time unloading clean dishes. She was blunt when I needed a better hairdresser, too, and found me just the right one.

We have always been very different. I left home at eighteen and didn't look back. Gigi never severed ties with our parents. After her marriage ended, she moved back into our parents' home with her two toddlers. When she later bought a house of her own, she chose one on the same street as Mom and Dad. Early on, she helped run one of our father's five restaurants, but found the hours punishing. She quit and went into teaching so she could spend every school holiday with her children. To me, that seemed to indicate a lack of ambition. I had always put career before family.

Still, I benefited from my sister's parenting expertise. As the mother of two children slightly older than mine, Gigi was ahead of me on the parental learning curve. She would tell me when to stop tying my boys' shoes, when to stop jumping up to refill their glasses of milk, when to stop packing their suitcases for them. She would admonish me by saying, "They're old enough!"

I am forever grateful that Gigi took care of our parents as they aged. She accompanied them to every doctor's appointment, and there were many, especially after Mom had a debilitating stroke and was later diagnosed with lung cancer. Though our two brothers lived in Montreal, the entire burden of care fell on my sister. She kept vigil at each operation. When Mom was recuperating, Gigi drove to the hospital three or four times a day to coax her to eat, brush her teeth and tuck her in at night. I flew to Montreal and did what I could. I cleaned the hospital toilet that Mom shared with three other patients. When the doctors suggested it would be better for her to move to an assisted-living residence, I helped scout out the best one. A lightning visit. An efficient look at three places. A quick decision.

But I didn't stick around. I lived in Toronto and I had to get back to work. When Mom objected to living in an institution, even a fancy one, I wasn't there to help her move back home. I wasn't there for when her weight dropped and her pain became chronic either. Still, I went to Montreal as often as I could, taking the boys to visit her during school holidays and summer vacations. I phoned her every week because she loved to talk about whatever book she was reading. I tried to contribute in other ways, too. I had made a career of asking tough questions, so I now assumed the awkward role of asking about her last wishes. Did she want to be resuscitated? Did she want a feeding tube? Did she want us to pull the plug? My sister didn't like me talking to Mom that way. And neither did Mom, who hesitated and then said slowly, "I don't want to die of dehydration." I persisted. What did she mean *exactly*? If she stopped breathing, should we try to revive her? Should we call an ambulance? Reluctantly, Mom told me only that she wanted a peaceful death.

Despite everything I did, it was no substitute for being there. I loved my mother but I didn't feel I could take time off work. Isn't that what everyone says? And then after supper one evening, Mom's heart gave out. Gigi screamed for Dad, who yelled for someone to call an ambulance. Mindful of Mom's last wishes, my sister burst into tears and refused. Her sixteen-year-old son, Will, caught between his mother, his grandfather and his dying grandmother, called 911. The paramedics worked on Mom, noisily. Gigi heard everything. From another room, she agonized over our mother's last wishes, but did not intervene. By the time the emergency workers put our mother's limp body onto a stretcher and into the ambulance, she had been dead for more than thirty minutes. My sister followed them to the hospital in her own car. By the time she had parked and found the right cubicle in the emergency room, the doctors had gotten Mom breathing again. My sister had the unbearable task of telling them to remove the life support.

From that instant, Gigi severed her relationship with me. She left the hospital that night, went back home and did not even phone me to say Mom had passed away. It was left up to my nephew, Will, to call me in the middle of the night. Using the Chinese words for maternal grandmother, he said, "Po Po died." I roused Norman and the boys, and we left Toronto at dawn. When we got to Montreal after five hours on the highway, I found the floor still strewn with syringes, ECG electrodes and packaging from the defibrillating paddles that had been used to shock her heart. I imagined my mother's ribs cracking as the paramedics thumped her chest.

My sister's grief was cataclysmic and exclusionary. That weekend, she shut herself inside our mother's bedroom and would not come out. For the next two years, she would not speak to me, refusing to take my calls, shunning me whenever I went to Montreal to visit Dad. At first, I was hurt especially because she had not called me herself about our mother's passing. As the weeks and months slipped by, my sister's rejection of me scalded. I wanted to call her and scream.

Colleen Parrish, who is married to my cousin, Ted, counseled patience. "Just wait. Your sister loves you." So I waited. What else could I do? I did not believe that our shattered relationship would ever heal. Nor did I know what I had done wrong. I searched for the reason my sister had cut me out of her life. Eventually, I concluded that I hadn't done anything, that I was completely innocent, that the rift was all her fault. Ironically, I heard through others that Gigi agreed, at least with the first part: I hadn't done anything.

Siblings always resent when one does more. Belatedly it dawned on me that my sister felt I had left the burden of Mom's care to her. (Our brothers weren't even in the equation.) In hindsight, I should have taken a leave of absence to be with Mom, but there was always another big story, another assignment, another deadline. Perhaps I had subconsciously absorbed the newsroom culture, a merciless environment where we avidly report on plane crashes and mayhem and mass murder. Two days after my mother was cremated, for instance, the editors assigned me a particularly controversial story. I do not recall the specifics, only that they were so eager for me in particular to handle it that when I demurred, the editor-in-chief personally called me at home. (When I apologized and explained I was temporarily unable to muster the requisite pit-bull instincts to do the story justice, he reluctantly backed off.)

Two years later, when my sister finally began accepting my calls, our conversations were brief and bloodless, centered on logistical information about Dad. Gigi remained remote. Typically and rather dysfunctionally, I tried to patch up the relationship using my journalistic skills. When her daughter, Alisha, applied to Columbia University and asked for my help, I eagerly edited her application essay even though I was sure she was bright enough to get in on her own merits. After Columbia accepted Alisha, my sister gradually thawed and we resumed diplomatic relations. She never mentioned our rift and neither did I. Perhaps she accepted who I was. More likely she simply resigned herself to my inability to change.

It was only much later, in the middle of my illness, that Gigi let slip what she thought of me at the time of our mother's death. By then we had grown so close that we talked almost daily, sometimes for hours at a time. "I didn't like you very much," she said offhandedly.

"You didn't like me?" My tone of genuine hurt made her laugh out loud.

"You were so selfish. You only thought about yourself."

I fell silent, thinking about what my sister had said. I concluded that she was mistaken. I wasn't selfish; I was merely driven. I was passionate about work. Any good reporter would always put the story first. But my sister saw my workaholism for what it was: an addiction, a sickness, a pathology. She saw the warning signs of depression long before I did. And that was why when I cracked, she understood. Not only did she understand, she came back to rescue me.

I arrived in Montreal on Thursday, September 14, 2006. It was twenty-four hours after the rampage and more than a dozen people were in serious or critical condition. Incredibly, there had been only one fatality, Anastasia De Sousa, the young woman into whom Gill had pumped eight extra bullets. As I had anticipated, the police had encircled Dawson College with yellow, plastic, do-not-cross-this-line tape. Like all the other journalists, I had to write a descriptive story without being able to enter the premises. Gigi showed me the area where one of her former students had been smoking a cigarette. "He was shot in the head," she said, pointing out the spot. "He's in critical condition now." She gestured to a wall of windows. "The atrium is straight ahead. The cafeteria is on the right."

Three years had passed since Mom's death. In the past twelve months we had slipped back, guardedly, into our old relationship, the one in which she chauffeured me from spot to spot and tried her best to help me when stories brought me to Montreal. On this occasion, she had picked me up at my hotel as soon as I arrived. Now we stood on the sidewalk outside Dawson while she told me what kind of food the cafeteria sold and where the vending machines and tables were. It was the quotidian detail I needed to set the scene for my newspaper's readers.

Kimveer Gill had shot twenty people. It could have been much worse, but two rookie police officers arrived by chance on a drug-related tip three minutes after he began shooting. Veteran cops might have waited for backup. The rookies drew their guns and rushed into the cafeteria. Gill stopped shooting. He grabbed the young man who had tried to pull De Sousa to safety and, using him as a human shield, backed into a corner near the vending machines. As students screamed and cowered under tables, one of the cops managed to wound Gill in the arm. At 12:48 P.M., six minutes after he entered Dawson, Gill committed suicide with a single shot to the head.

After Gigi finished explaining Dawson's layout, she drove me back to my hotel. On the car radio, a talk-show host was saying that all three of Canada's campus shootings had occurred in Montreal. *That's right*, I thought with surprise. *But why?* That evening Gigi and I dropped by to see Jay Bryan, a friend and columnist at the *Gazette*. I mentioned what I'd heard on the radio. "A lot of people are saying: why does this always happen in Quebec?" Jay said. "Three doesn't mean anything. But three out of three in Quebec means something."

Like epidemiologists who look for patterns in the outbreak and spread of diseases, reporters also seek meaning in chaos—except we must do so on deadline. Three out of three was statistically meaningless, but not in a business where we grasp for any pattern. For journalists, three is a magic number: it's a trend.

Back in my hotel room, I considered the fact that Gill was the son of immigrants from India. I remembered another campus shooting in

Montreal had also involved an immigrant, a Russian named Valery Fabrikant, who had killed four colleagues at Concordia University. In the third and bloodiest campus shooting, Marc Lépine had murdered fourteen women at École Polytechnique, an engineering school affiliated with Université de Montréal. That rampage had occurred nearly seventeen years earlier, in 1989, when I was working overseas as the *Globe*'s Beijing correspondent. Dimly I remembered there had been something unusual about Lépine. I couldn't put my finger on it, but before I went to sleep, I sent an email query to the newspaper: check Lépine's background.

The next morning, I received the answer. Lépine was born Gamil Gharbi, the son of a Muslim businessman from Algeria. Suddenly, I had a trend: all three shooters came from immigrant stock. What were the odds of that in a province dominated by francophones and a smaller anglophone minority? An hour later when the national editor called to find out my angle, I mentioned that none of Quebec's school shooters were francophone or anglophone. I said my story would explore the idea of immigrants, ethnicity and alienation.

"Fabulous," she said.

I spent the morning interviewing Gigi's office-mate, Pina, and her son. He told me he had been moving between classes, listening to his iPod, oblivious to the gunfire and had almost stumbled upon the killer in the atrium. Luckily, a bleeding young woman had rushed past, screaming at him to run.

By the time I finished my interviews and research, only three hours remained before deadline. I wrote quickly, leading with the interviews with Pina and her son. In the fifteenth paragraph I inserted the analysis my editor had asked for:

What many outsiders don't realize is how alienating the decades-long linguistic struggle has been in the once-cosmopolitan city. It hasn't just taken a toll on long-time anglophones; it's affected immigrants, too.

To be sure, the shootings in all three cases were carried out by mentally disturbed individuals. But what is also true is that in all three cases, the perpetrator was not pure laine, the argot for a "pure" francophone. Elsewhere, to talk of racial "purity" is repugnant. Not in Quebec

I knew that invoking the term, *pure laine*, would touch a nerve. It means "pure wool," and is used on sweater labels in France, but in my home province it's slang for old-stock Quebeckers. I, for instance, could never be considered *pure laine*, even though my family has lived in Quebec for a century. In the soul-searching following the Dawson shootings, it seemed the right moment to raise the issue of blood and belonging. So I added:

> *To be sure, Mr. Lépine hated women, Mr. Fabrikant hated his engineering colleagues and Mr. Gill hated everyone. But all of them had been marginalized, in a society that valued* pure laine.

By 6 P.M., I emailed the first two thousand words to the newspaper. By 7:30 P.M., I filed the final one thousand words. Exhausted and starved, I headed for dinner at an Indian restaurant with Gigi, my former colleague, Jay, and his wife, Laura. We were munching on pappadums and about to order our meal when the national editor called. She had almost finished editing the story.

"We love this *pure laine* stuff," she said. "Can you give us more?"

I stopped munching and flipped through my notebook. I had been high on adrenaline for twenty-four hours and was now brain-dead. Otherwise I might have remembered the uproar after a Quebec premier complained that the province's "white race" was not having enough babies. I might have mentioned the hit television show, *Pure Laine*. I might have reminded her of the province's suicide rate, the highest in Canada. I didn't even remember— and neither did the national editor—the well-known fact that Quebec's net outflow of immigrants was the highest in Canada.

At that moment I could find nothing more to add.

"Sorry," I told her, closing my notebook. "That's all I've got."

The next day the *Globe* ran the story under a banner headline. And then the backlash began. In a stunningly short time, I went from being a reporter who could pull off a three-thousand-word feature in one day to someone who could no longer write at all.

CHAPTER 3

L'Affaire Wong

"Sick fucking communist cunt."

That Monday I received hundreds of hate emails. "Piece of shit," "bitch," "stupid cunt," "retarded," "pathetic," "perverted," "bigoted," "you suck," "fucking asshole," "you poor cunt," "racist pig," "idiot," "stupid," "crap," "garbage," "vomit." One called my children "half-breeds." Several wrote, "Go back to China." Another lobbed this: "Your parents were immigrants."

A few were unwittingly prescient. "Consult a psychiatrist," one advised. Another said, "I hope you lose your job."

In an interview with *The New York Times Sunday Magazine*, the film director and author Nora Ephron once said, "Any catastrophe is good material for a writer." She's right, especially in the case of journalists. When we are abused, we split into two. We feel as bad as anyone, but we also record the action and our own reaction. Even as I felt the sting of the emails, it occurred to me that the onslaught might make an ironic follow-up: a racist backlash on a minority reporter from Quebec for suggesting racism alienated minorities in Quebec. I began taking notes. I rated the emails and voice mails on a yellow legal pad. Ten percent were supportive, 15 percent were neutral and 75 percent were vitriolic.

That was Monday. I didn't know it at the time, but the *Globe* had already invited an editor at *La Presse*, a French-language newspaper in Quebec, to write a commentary about me. It ran on Tuesday, under the headline: "*Pure laine is pure nonsense.*" More emails poured into my in-box. After tabulating several hundred, I gave up and saved them to read later. After all, I had to concentrate on my next story. A couple of days earlier at the Toronto International Film Festival, the actor Sean Penn had lit up during a press conference in a no-smoking meeting room at the Sutton Place Hotel. The paparazzi snapped incriminating photos. Shock and horror ensued. My boss, the deputy managing editor of features, assigned me to personally test the city's anti-smoking bylaw.

"Make sure you smoke where there are police."

A non-smoker, I duly bought a pack of cigarettes. With a photographer in tow, I hit ten spots including, of course, the Sutton Place Hotel. One coffee-shop owner called the police. A restaurant manager yelled at me and kicked me out. Scandalized cops at the Ontario Court of Appeal ordered me to butt out. The hotel concierge ejected me and ostentatiously spritzed the lobby with air freshener.

That night, I went home reeking of tobacco smoke and drained from risking arrest ten times in one day. I barely noticed that my newspaper had published a letter from the premier of Quebec calling my report "a disgrace." An editorial on the same page, written by the editor-in-chief himself, suggested there had been "no evidence" for my *pure laine* analysis. In Ottawa, the Parliament of Canada passed a unanimous motion demanding that I apologize "to the people of Quebec for the offensive remarks."

I felt somewhat chagrined, but not terribly so. As Harold Evans, former editor of the *Sunday Times* and *The Times* of London, wrote, "Independent reporting has a history of provoking denunciation." I figured that if I wasn't provoking a debate, I wasn't doing my job.

But that week the *Globe* kept publishing letters—thirteen in all—under headings like "Dangerous clichés," "Narrow-minded analysis" and "Absurd viewpoint." In Quebec, the media began calling the event "*l'affaire Wong*." They noted that the *Globe* appeared to be backing away from its reporter and its story. The steady drumbeat of attention triggered more hate email. "Consider yourself lucky that no one has yet been alienated enough to go postal on you."

As the number of emails exploded—I got hundreds and then thousands— it did not occur to the newspaper or me that someone else should screen them for me. So I kept reading the hate emails and tabulating them, and I kept feeling worse. In a way the onslaught was reminiscent of China's Cultural Revolution where victims would stand, heads bowed, while others spewed invective, hate and spittle. Or perhaps it was more like being pilloried in medieval stocks. Was I the village miscreant, locked head and hands in a wooden frame while others hurled rotting vegetables at me?

No, I thought, this was merely an Internet stoning. Of course I would be fine. *Sticks and stones may break my bones, but words can never hurt me.* Yet I was surprised how much words did hurt. Had I always been so sensitive? Or had my work environment changed? When I first began working as a journalist, readers would send in letters to the editor the old-fashioned way. It took effort and money to write thoughts down on paper, address an envelope, look up the postal code, stick on a stamp and drop the letter in an actual mailbox. Now people just typed fast and smacked the send button.

As the furor intensified, other media began besieging me with interview requests. I turned them down because I didn't want to become the news, any more than I already was. The senior editors agreed. "If we keep our heads down, it will blow over very quickly. We don't want to fan the flames," advised Sylvia Stead, the *Globe*'s deputy editor, who was in charge of legal matters and the most powerful woman in the newsroom. My editors and I were on the same page. We were a team. It was all of us on the inside against the crazies on the outside.

On Thursday evening, I was finishing up my puff piece when a colleague in the Montreal bureau phoned me at home. He had also been grappling with the fallout from my Dawson story and now, as part of his bureau duties, he was letting me know that an extremist website had launched an attack on my family. *Le Québécois* had labeled my eighty-six-year-old father a "convicted criminal" and said that he had served thirty-one months in prison for an immigration scam. My colleague added that the website also was calling for a boycott of my family's restaurant, Bill Wong's Inc. This is how Patrick Bourgeois, the website's editor, put it: "Perhaps they try to take revenge against pure laine Québecois stock in selling cat or rat disguised as chicken."

Given the virulent response to my Dawson article, I had no doubt there would be a boycott. I began to shake. I had maintained my equilibrium all week, but now my family was under attack and it was entirely my fault. I didn't yet know that one symptom of depression is all-consuming guilt. I didn't yet know that narcissism, another symptom, intensifies the guilt. *I* had written about the Dawson shootings and therefore *I* had ruined my father's good name and jeopardized the family business.

My colleague in the Montreal bureau was still on the phone. "Of course it's not your father," he continued. "It's another man, in his forties, with the same name. I know because I wrote the original story."

I asked my colleague what I should do.

"Your father has deep pockets," he said, ending the call.

Newsroom culture is like that. There's no time for handholding. Everyone is on a deadline. I'm sure my colleague in Montreal had no idea how it felt on my end, but I felt utterly abandoned. The racial attack shattered me. Looking back, I believe this was the exact moment I began my descent into depression. I let out a scream and burst into tears. Ben and Sam came running. Not knowing what had happened, they wrapped me in hugs—the way I had done when they were toddlers and they had bumped their knees.

Stir-frying rodent flesh is an outlandish allegation, and one that reflects on the accuser. But I was not rational at that moment. And unless you have experienced racism, it is hard to explain its corrosiveness. You feel frightened and violated and impotent all at once. When race is perceived to be a factor, the hurt from almost any slight, even an innocent, unintended one, can last a lifetime. Before she married my father, my mother worked as an operating-room nurse in Montreal for Wilder Penfield, the renowned neurosurgeon. Mom had loved her job and love to reminisce about how she could slap the correct scalpel into his palm before he could ask for it. She also never forgot that she was the only team member he had not once invited to his Westmount home.

Ben was four when we went sightseeing in Gravenhurst, a bucolic Ontario town. At one point, we stopped at a park where several white boys, all about ten years old, were playing. I was preoccupied with Sam when I suddenly noticed the older boys had left and Ben was missing. I found him crouching under a slide. Only after much coaxing, he told me that when he had approached the boys, one of them had pointed to a discarded soft drink can, in which a wasp was crawling out of the opening, and said, "Hey, Chinese boy. Kick that." Now, at nineteen, Ben remembers every detail of that day. The weather was sunny. The bigger kid was "chubby, with light hair." He can still visualize the soft drink can and the wasp that the other boy hoped would sting him.

Perhaps it is remarkable that, until now no one had attacked me for my race in all the years and in all the places I had worked as a journalist. Certainly it had never been an issue at the *Globe* where I was the only visible minority among fifty-eight columnists listed on the newspaper's website. That evening, when I calmed down, I went to read the website for *Le Québécois* myself. I vaguely remembered hearing about it a year earlier when it had pilloried the first black woman to be appointed governor-general of Canada. As I read the diatribe against my family's restaurant, I thought about how Dad had opened the restaurant in Montreal nearly half a century earlier. I thought about my grandfather, who came to Canada in 1880 to help build the Canadian Pacific Railway. I don't know what it was like for him then, except that in 1883 *The New York Times* was soberly asking the question, "Do Chinese eat rats?"

I had not expected to hear that Yellow-Peril calumny in *my* lifetime. When I finished reading *Le Québécois*, I phoned the *Globe*'s libel lawyer. He said he would shut down the web page for me, but he needed the name, address and phone number of the site's legal owner. In desperation I called another colleague in the Montreal bureau who had written a couple of stories about *Le Québécois* a few months earlier. Fighting my tears, I explained what had just happened. Could she help me find the owner? Like my other colleague in the Montreal bureau, she had no idea what I had been through that week. "I'm in a restaurant having dinner," she said, shouting over the din. "I don't remember anything about them. You can look it up."

I hung up and burst into tears again. It felt like a betrayal when my coworkers told me: "You can look it up," or "Your father has deep pockets." Normally I have no problem digging up information, but suddenly I didn't think I could manage to find anything on my own. Still crying, I phoned my friend, Talin Vartanian, a radio producer at the Canadian Broadcasting Corporation. "I'll be right over," she promised. She arrived within minutes and immediately sat down to call her media contacts in Montreal. Meanwhile Ben suggested I capture the web page for evidence. When I looked at him helplessly, my sixteen-year-old did it for me. Then he began translating the French text into English for the *Globe*'s lawyer.

All this time, my husband, Norman, had been hovering in the background. I hadn't paid much attention when he sat down and began typing on my laptop. He opened the command interpreter, typed a special code and then the domain name for *Le Québécois*.

"I've got it," he said calmly.

"How did you do *that*?" I said, amazed, staring over his shoulder at the computer screen. The registration information had popped up—the name, address and home phone number of the website owner and more.

"When I worked for a computer company in the mid-1990s," he said, "I helped develop a piece of software that lets you access information from behind a firewall."

Whatever *that* meant. I had never paid much attention to Norman's work. He is a systems engineer. Although he had steadfastly supported my career, following me from Beijing to New York to Montreal to Boston to Toronto and back to Beijing again, I had scarcely reciprocated. In fact, whenever I had insomnia, my solution was to nudge him awake and ask about his doctoral thesis. He would become *animated*, well, not quite animated, but he would start talking at length about parallel programming languages and the semantics of shared variables. As he droned on, I would fall deeply asleep, leaving *him* wide-awake.

I justified this spousal abuse as feminism. It was a philosophy I first embraced as a university freshman when I devoured books by Betty Friedan, Gloria Steinem and Simone de Beauvoir. When Norman and I met in 1975, I was twenty-four and studying at Peking University for my second degree in Chinese history. He was nine years older, from New York City, working in Beijing as a translator for a government propaganda magazine.

He had come to China as an American draft dodger. In fact, he was the only American draft dodger to take refuge there during the Vietnam War. He was tall and thin (and still is). He spoke fluent, unaccented Chinese (and still does). He hated cooking and wearing ties, but liked to eat and could fix a broken lamp or leaky bicycle tire. I fell in love.

We were opposites. I was Type A. He was off the alphabet. He was shy, easy-going, reticent, forgetful, slow and always late. I was extroverted, tightly wound, impatient, outspoken, organized and punctual. I was extravagantly emotional. He was phlegmatic and calm, except when he emitted the occasional deep sigh or shockingly explosive guffaw.

Even before we got married, I was sure I could improve him. When we were dating, for instance, I tired of being the one who always made the arrangements so I gave him a test. "I don't know if you are serious, but I am," I announced one day over a bowl of dumplings in Beijing. "You have to call me three times within an unspecified period of time or it's over."

In my mind, I gave him three weeks to convince me he loved me. Norman managed to rouse himself to phone three times in two weeks. And so we got married. Despite abundant nagging about doing things faster or multi-tasking or being more decisive, to my utter surprise and dismay, he didn't change. And neither did I. In restaurants, I wished he would flag down the waiter for me. I wished he would organize something fun for us to do on Saturday night. I wished he would dream up at least one outing a month for the boys. But he seemed constitutionally unable to do such things. Over thirty years of marriage, I admit that these minor annoyances began to dull my love for him. I now see what a walking contradiction I was: a feminist who wanted her husband to take charge—but only occasionally and only when she told him to.

That Thursday I stayed up all night dealing with the website. Using information Norman and Talin unearthed, the *Globe*'s lawyer tracked down the owner of *Le Québécois* at his home north of Montreal and threatened him with a lawsuit unless he removed the page attacking my family. By Friday morning, the page had vanished and a correction and apology had appeared.

After a sleepless night, I phoned my father. I dreaded telling him the website had called him a crook and a jailbird, but I had to warn him about the potential boycott. "Don't worry," said Dad, who is blind in one eye, deaf in one ear and isn't easily agitated. His only brush with the law had been a ticket, thirty years earlier, for driving without a seat belt. The last time I remember him getting upset was during the 1995 referendum over Quebec's independence. He had voted, like a record 94 percent of his fellow citizens, and then paced all night while the tally was counted. The final nail-biting result: 49.42 percent for separation versus 50.58 percent against.

Dad and I had watched the results, and kept watching as Premier Jacques Parizeau addressed a roomful of tearful supporters. "We were so close to a country," he told them. "It's true that we have been defeated—but basically—by what? By money and the ethnic vote."

Dad had flinched at that. By "money," did Parizeau mean my father, a successful businessman who once owned five restaurants in Montreal? Was my father one of those despised "ethnics"? And would he always be one, even though he was born in Quebec a decade before Parizeau?

The attack by Le Québécois was only the beginning. The next morning a caricature in Le Devoir, a respected Quebec daily, showed me opening fortune cookies to decode the news. The sketch depicted me with buckteeth and Coke-bottle-bottom glasses, an echo of the anti-Japanese stereotypes of the Second World War. My race was irrelevant to my reporting. To my surprise, my eyes filled with tears.

It was Friday, the end of a horrible week. The Globe's editor-in-chief summoned me to a meeting. Edward Greenspon was waiting in his office, a glassed-in box on the edge of the newsroom. Shakily I took a seat across from him. Without preamble, he pushed a copy of my Dawson article across the table. He had circled the offending paragraphs with a black marker. "This should have been taken out, or it should have been labeled analysis," he said, pointing to the marked passages. "I want you to go through this, line by line, and tell me if there's anything you have changed your mind about."

Startled, I asked if he had read the story before publication. He pulled the newspaper back across the table and scanned the article. "I remember reading about the daycare," he said slowly. "That section comes after pure laine, so I guess I did."

Greenspon had become the top editor at the Globe after a solid career of reporting on the political scene in Ottawa. He understood news. He also understood the complicated situation in Quebec. I was puzzled why he asking me to justify something he had already vetted himself. It turned out that he was planning to write about me in his Saturday commentary.

"Tomorrow my column is going to have two things, one positive and one negative. You're the negative. I'm going to say you erred."

I thought our strategy was to keep our heads down. Hadn't his deputy told me it was best not to "fan the flames"? Perhaps the editor-in-chief hadn't heard about the caricature in that morning's *Le Devoir*. Perhaps he didn't know that the previous night an extremist website had slandered my father and called for a boycott of my family's restaurant. I told him I felt a line had been crossed when a reporter's family or race was attacked. I mentioned the many interview requests I had received. I asked if he could accept one of them and use the opportunity to condemn these attacks on my family and me.

"I can't control the message if I do interviews [with other media]," Greenspon said, shaking his head. "I prefer to write in the paper. I can control it that way."

I felt utterly abandoned. In the past, I had always had the unwavering support of my paper whenever I had been savaged for my work. Not this time, it seemed.

I was despondent when I returned to my desk and checked the latest hate email. Someone named Claude Perron wrote:

Is it true your father spent 31 months in prison for exploiting Asian immigrants? Is it true your father's restaurant was condemned for filth? Is it dirty in your home? Is it true that Chinese food is dirty? Is it true that you don't wash your ass?

Philippe Mark emailed in French: "Do you speak French? I expect not. You should return to the country of your origin. I will join the boycott of the Wong restaurant."

The cartoon in *Le Devoir* prompted France Gervais to write: "That is not a caricature of you, but exactly the way you look. You have slanted eyes and you have buckteeth. You are Chinese. What's the problem?"

Another emailer sneered: "What you want—you were born with buckteeth?"

Andre Valiquette: "Hey Wong, I have seen the caricature and your picture. You are much uglier in real life ... Bitch."

Sebastien Boisvert: "The real problem ... is how ugly you are."

Mario Gagné: "Go back to barbarian China."

Suddenly, I had had enough. Now that my newspaper was about to criticize me in print, yet again, I would no longer be silenced. The policy of "keeping our heads down" seemed entirely one-sided. Everyone else was allowed to speak out except me. My newspaper had made it clear that it wouldn't defend my family or me, so I would have to respond to the attacks myself.

I went back downstairs to the editor-in-chief's office. I told him I had decided to accept a few interviews. "Why don't you write a commentary for *La Presse*?" Greenspon said. "I can arrange that." Normally, I would have agreed, but I was hollowed out. I had slept badly for days. I did not have the energy left to write a response. What I did not yet realize was that I couldn't write anything at all.

I told the editor-in-chief that I could only handle *being* interviewed. I couldn't write something myself. Perhaps that's when he noticed how upset I was. At any rate, he felt a rehearsal was in order. He sat me down on a couch in his deputy's office and role-played a television host lobbing questions at me. It felt surreal.

Late that afternoon, I accepted two interviews, one print and one radio. On its national newscast, a CBC radio reporter asked me why both the premier of Quebec and the prime minister of Canada had criticized me. For any journalist, that was a no brainer. "Because they need votes," I said, "in Quebec."

CHAPTER 4

A Threat Close to Home

What is it like to fall apart without realizing you are falling apart? On Saturday I fetched the paper from the mat outside my front door and turned to the editor-in-chief's column. By now I was hypersensitive and my eyes flew past the words of praise—"Jan Wong, an extraordinarily talented feature writer ... the piece was exceptionally moving ... it captured the humanity beautifully..." Instead I focused on the criticism. Greenspon described it as "the worst of weeks for *The Globe and Mail*." He wrote that I had ventured into the "sensitive territory" of ethnic and linguistic relations in a province that has "struggled to maintain its identity." He continued:

> *The response was swift and furious. Quebeckers of all stripes were deeply insulted. They felt the depiction was outmoded in the cosmopolitan reality of modern Montreal and that any connection to past language battles was spurious and contrived....*
>
> *While we feel the reaction to the article has been disproportionate—including personal attacks on Jan and her family—in hindsight, the paragraphs were clearly opinion and not reporting and should have been removed from the story...*

Reading this now, several years later, my editor-in-chief's words don't seem all that terrible. But it was a measure of how close I was to a complete breakdown that I saw only the criticism, and it devastated me. Even in calmer times, however, it's hard to explain to those who don't make their living tackling controversy how critical it is for journalists to have their boss at their back. We constantly rush toward danger. We take risks. We deliver messages people do not always want to hear, hence the common reflex: shoot the messenger.

Journalists never do stories alone. An entire editing team supports us—checking spelling, grammar and punctuation, weighing the choice of words, the logic, the accuracy, the fairness and balance. Nothing gets into the newspaper without having been vetted by several sets of eyes. The result is an unwritten newsroom code: if the paper prints the story, the editor-in-chief stands behind it. For a journalist, betrayal by your own can be devastating. Ten years earlier, Gary Webb, a Pulitzer Prize-winning reporter for the *San Jose Mercury News*, wrote a three-part investigative series linking CIA-backed Contras in Nicaragua to the crack-cocaine epidemic in Los Angeles. The series got 1.3 million hits a day on the newspaper's website and at first the *Mercury News* reveled in the attention.

But eight months later, after the White House counterattacked and major news outlets, including the *Washington Post* and the *New York Times*, tried to debunk the series, the *Mercury News* wobbled. "I believe that we fell short at every step of our process," the executive editor wrote in a letter to readers. Webb was reassigned to a suburban bureau one hundred and fifty miles from his home. The commute was arduous and the demotion humiliating. He eventually quit the paper. In 2004, he committed suicide. Since his death, two other major newspapers, including the *Los Angeles Times*, one of his initial naysayers, have validated his conclusions.

In his Saturday column, my editor-in-chief did not tell *Globe* readers he had read my Dawson story before publication. Instead he wrote:

I can offer several explanations as to how the editorial quality control process sometimes breaks down on tight deadlines during grueling weeks. But none are germane. The fact is they did, which is ultimately my responsibility. We regret that we allowed these words to get into a reported article.

Through the years I had often written about corporations and corporate backpedaling, but somehow I had convinced myself that newspapers were different. I guess I had drunk the Kool-Aid. I naively thought we would embody the ideals we championed in our pages. I thought newsroom managers would behave better. In the end, they were just managers.

That weekend, I hardly slept. Stead, the deputy editor phoned me that Sunday to tell me, again, "We don't want to fan the flames." She wanted to know my reaction to Greenspon's column. I told her he had read my article before it was published. She said she was sure the controversy was subsiding.

It was not. The media in Quebec translated the editor-in-chief's column into French. They lavished more newsprint on *l'affaire Wong*. They discussed why the Globe was apologizing and why it "regretted" the story. My family's restaurant, which my older brother was now running, began receiving abusive phone calls. *Le Québécois*, which had withdrawn the libel of my father, now published a cartoon of me, finger on chin, contemplating three Chinese take-out food containers, variously labeled "cat," "dog" and "Québécois." The thought bubble above my head: "What shall I have for lunch today? A difficult choice."

Early on Monday a radio station in Montreal called about my editor-in-chief's column. The morning-show host asked me why he had backed away from the Dawson story. I said I didn't know why, especially as he had read it ahead of publication. Afterward, I sent an email to my editor-in-chief expressing my disappointment in his Saturday column. I said his response had been "inherently untruthful" because the quality control process, as he put it, had *not* broken down—I had filed my story on time and he himself had cleared it.

Fourteen minutes later, at 11:16 A.M., Greenspon sent me a response from his BlackBerry. He said I had misread what he had written. "The system did break down. Editors, in addition to reporters, make judgments. In this case, we—and I include myself—should have seen this was an unknowable thesis embedded in a (very well) reported story. The point is not ultimately the reaction, but the mix of words.... I came to this conclusion the following morning, well before any reaction."

Greenspon added that he was out of the country and would leave the matter with Stead, his deputy. "My impression is this has blown over. I would be careful not to fuel it further."

At 11:49 A.M., Stead sent me an email ordering me not to speak any more about the Dawson story. "As I said to you on the phone yesterday, we don't want this to bleed into this week as well. I appreciate very much that you have kept your head down on this. I think it is done and we want it to be, so you are not to talk to any media about the story or the reaction to the story without first speaking to me."

For the first time in my career as a journalist, I had been silenced. I felt myself disintegrating. The rest of that day, I did little except read more hate email. After work, I attended a reception at the Toronto headquarters of the Daily Bread Food Bank, which was giving me its annual public-service award for an undercover series I had recently written about working as a maid. To my intense embarrassment, during my brief acceptance remarks on stage, I began to cry.

The next morning, I had a meeting on another matter with the new vice-president of human resources. To my surprise, Phillip Crawley, the *Globe's* publisher and CEO, was waiting in her office. He was livid. "You were told last week and on Sunday not to talk to the media, and you talked."

"That's not true," I said, too startled to explain how the strategy had changed on Friday and how the editor-in-chief himself had coached me on how to handle a television interview.

"You have hurt our brand in Quebec," Crawley continued, adding that he was launching an internal investigation. The publisher nodded at the HR vice-president, who had stood up behind her desk. "She will be in charge of the investigation."

After he left, I burst into tears. I couldn't stop sobbing. I felt panic, alarm and utter desolation. It had been thirteen days since I had had a proper night's sleep. The HR executive, a woman I had never met, wordlessly handed me a tissue. I wasn't afraid of an investigation because I had done nothing wrong. But I couldn't understand why Crawley, who ran the business side of the newspaper, was getting involved. I told the HR vice-president that I would forward to her all relevant email. She nodded. Again, she said nothing.

I helped myself to another tissue and wiped my tears. Then I hurried off to a features meeting. I felt like fleeing. Perhaps I would get a travel assignment that would take me away from all this strife. At the meeting, Cathrin Bradbury, the deputy managing editor of features had no inkling how sensitive the Dawson story had become. She had loved my initial feature and indeed wanted me to travel—back to Montreal for an exclusive interview with the family of the killer. I shuddered and declined.

After the features meeting, I dropped by the office of John Stackhouse, the business editor. I would soon be reporting to him as the new Asia-Pacific correspondent, covering economics and politics in China, India and Japan. A week earlier he had determined that my first trip would be to India. He had advised me I would be leaving within six to eight weeks. Suddenly, I couldn't leave soon enough and asked him if we could nail down a specific date. To my astonishment, Stackhouse told me I had misunderstood. I didn't have the job after all.

"We're still interviewing other candidates," he said.

It had been twenty-four hours since I had challenged my editor-in-chief about his column and only an hour since the publisher had chastised me for "hurting the brand." Call me stupid, but I didn't make the connection. Instead, I was bewildered. The Asia-Pacific assignment was a perfect fit for my skills, experience and interests. I had already had several meetings with the business editor over my new assignment. I wondered if I was losing my mind.

In a state of shock, I went home and told Norman that the Asia-Pacific job wasn't mine after all. When I had first applied for the posting, we had talked it over at length because the position was based out of Toronto and he was concerned about the heavy travel required. But when I got it, he had congratulated me. Now my husband said that I could not possibly have misunderstood a promotion. Suddenly I felt like Joseph K., the protagonist in Kafka's *The Trial*. A fragment of the famous opening line came to mind: "... for without having done anything wrong he was arrested one fine morning."

What had I done wrong?

I called Gigi to tell her the bad news. Unlike me, she immediately connected the dots. She said that it must be some kind of punishment for Dawson. She tried to console me. "It would have taken you away too much. Ben and Sam need you."

That night, unable to sleep for what seemed like the umpteenth night, I wrote the publisher a brief note. I explained how difficult the previous week had been for my family and me. I said I thought it best for the newspaper to move on. The next morning I emailed my note and dropped off a copy with his secretary. At my desk, I continued reading emails. I thought it was part of my job. I didn't understand the toll processing hateful messages takes on the recipient. Every time someone called me "bitch" or "cunt" or "slanty-eyed," it had the corrosive effect Andrew Solomon describes in *The Noonday Demon*. Each new bit of venom ate away at my soul.

After several hours of this, I took a break and went downstairs to the library, taking some snail mail with me so I could multi-task in case the librarian was busy. She was indeed on the phone. While I waited, I opened a plain manila envelope addressed to me by hand. It had no return address, but the sender had written across the front: "Personal and confidential." Inside was a two-page letter, typed entirely in capitals.

"I KNOW WHERE YOU LIVE."

"Oh my goodness," said the librarian, looking over my shoulder. "You'd better put that down. Call security."

A guard answered on the first ring.

"I think I just got a death threat," I said, almost apologetically. Inside I was breaking into a thousand little pieces, but it seemed if I was polite, if I kept my voice low, I could hold it all together. While I waited for the guard to arrive, I continued to open other mail. One envelope contained a formal complaint to the Quebec Press Council about my Dawson story. Next I opened a small package containing two books I'd written on China. I felt better. *Someone wants me to autograph them.*

The librarian gasped as the books fell apart in chunks. They had been cleanly sawn in half with a power tool.

The security guard appeared. He donned a pair of latex gloves and took the threatening letter from me. "We didn't want to tell you, but an envelope arrived for you yesterday," he said. "It was either excrement or some kind of substance. The mailroom guys handled it."

My throat tightened. The guard examined the death threat and the manila envelope it came in. "I'm going to take this down to the security office and call the police," he said.

I wanted to hug him, the first person at my workplace who seemed to be on my side. My time in the stocks was ending.

In investigative-journalist mode, I headed straight to the mailroom to talk to the clerk. He confirmed that he had handled the item, but wasn't sure if it was excrement or something else.

"We already threw it out," he said. "It might have been blood."

Blood.

Suddenly I heard myself being paged. "Jan Wong, call security."

I hurried to a phone.

"I'm sorry," said the security guard, sounding embarrassed. "It looks like you'll have to call the police yourself."

Surely there was some misunderstanding. Why wouldn't security call the police for me? I ran down the hall to the security office. The chief of security was standing at the counter. He repeated what the security guard had told me: I had to phone the police myself.

"Could I use your phone?" I asked. I didn't actually *mean* I wanted to use his phone. I just didn't know what else to say. Something strange was happening to me. I didn't think I could manage a phone call. Much later, when I read *The Noonday Demon*, I understood. Solomon notes how preposterous breakdowns are. He describes lying in bed and crying because he was too frightened to take a shower, while at the same time knowing that showers are not scary.

I routinely made dozens of cold calls a day as part of my job. But at that moment I couldn't even articulate my inability to make a phone call. Suddenly, it seemed vitally important that the security office phone the police on my behalf. Anything else symbolized more betrayal. Everything was riding on this phone call, at least to me. I was in such a confused state that when I asked the chief of security if I could make the call *from* his office, I thought he would figure out that was code for: *please help me, please call for me.*

The chief of security did not understand the secret code. Why would he? Like every security guy in the world, he had not been hired for his sensitivity. He nodded with some exasperation and told me the number to call. I managed to punch the right digits. My voice shaking, I spoke briefly to the police, who said they would send someone over. "Can you wait there?" the officer said.

I could not. All at once I couldn't bear being at work another minute. My heart was thumping. My mouth was dry. I heard myself telling the police I was unable to wait for them. "Then call us after you get home," the police officer said.

I hung up the phone.

"You'll need to show them this," the chief of security said, handing me the threatening letter. I noticed that he wasn't wearing latex gloves.

"What about fingerprints?"

"Don't worry," he said. "This letter already has so many fingerprints on it."

I hesitated to touch it with my bare hands, but his arm was outstretched. I took the letter. I waited for him to offer me a ride home or make other arrangements. I knew that whenever reporters get credible death threats, they are typically sent to a safe place—a hotel or someone else's home. If the situation is judged serious enough, bodyguards are hired, too. Once again, the head of security seemed unable to understand the code. He stared at me. I stared back. And without another word, I returned to my desk.

My throat was so parched I felt I could no longer speak. I did not tell my editors I was leaving. I did not talk to a single colleague. Instead I stuffed the threatening letter into my backpack and slung it over my shoulders. As I walked out of the building, I thought I could feel the letter burning through the fabric, searing my back.

Bewilderment sharpened my distress. I couldn't explain anything that had happened in the past two weeks. A decade earlier when I got a threat at work, the company had immediately called the police. Why wouldn't my newspaper report it this time? What had I done wrong? Had I missed some warning signs? It was like asking the students who had gone to Dawson that day why someone had stormed their school. They hadn't seen the attack coming. No one ever does.

It did not occur to me to take a taxi or to call my husband. Instead, I scurried out the newsroom's back exit, which led to the *Globe*'s rooftop parking lot and a ramp down to the street. As I fled past the parked cars, I couldn't help remembering how an investigative reporter in Montreal had been shot five times in *his* newspaper's parking lot, one day after his story on biker gangs had been published. I glanced up at the abandoned sock factory next to the ramp. *A perfect spot for a sniper.* On the subway platform, I scanned the faces of the other passengers. To my relief, none looked to me like a killer.

Norman was surprised when I arrived home in the middle of the day. A few months earlier he had lost his job. Being out of work had never fazed him. He loved computers, but unlike me he had never defined himself through his work. He had already been laid off half a dozen times, beginning when the high-tech sector had nosedived in the 1990s. The loss of one job never seemed to affect his self-esteem. He would use the down time to keep up with his field, reading thick textbooks with titles like *Beautiful Code: Leading Programmers Explain How They Think* and *Operating Systems: Design and Implementation*. He always found another software job.

The first few times my husband was laid off, I had partly blamed him. Then I grew irritated as he sat, day after day, quietly reading in the flowered wing chair by the living room window. Now for the first time I was glad he was home. I showed him the letter and said I hadn't finished reading it. Would he look it over? He immediately agreed, but when he hesitated to touch it, I heard myself repeating what the head of security had told me. "Another set of fingerprints won't matter," I said.

I phoned the police as I had been instructed. "Is the threat imminent?" asked the officer who answered. The question threw me. What was "imminent"? I glanced through our brand-new windows, installed one week earlier. No one seemed to be lurking in the garden.

"I don't know. He says he's got a gun and he's going to kill me and he knows where I live."

"We'll be there soon."

After I hung up, my teeth began chattering. I suddenly felt very cold. *In The Year of Magical Thinking*, Joan Didion writes that she was always freezing in the months after her husband died. I didn't realize then that stress impairs circulation, a reason emergency crews hand out blankets to accident victims whether or not they have been injured. For the next two years, I was surprised to find that my feet were always icy. I would need a hot water bottle to fall asleep, even at the height of a summer heat wave.

As I waited for the police I wrapped myself in a blanket. It was late afternoon. I had not eaten or drunk anything since breakfast. I rarely miss a meal, but now the thought of food made me nauseous. Stress, in addition to impairing circulation, floods the body with adrenalin, which shuts down the digestive system so you can focus all your energy on fight or flight. Too much adrenalin can also make you throw up, hence my feeling of nausea.

At first, I didn't understand the evolutionary connection between adrenalin and nausea. Then I happened upon an exhibit at the Natural History Museum in London that showed that, when in danger, the South American black vulture reflexively vomits up the contents of its stomach to make itself lighter—and swifter—in flight.

I sat alone on the chintz couch in my living room and attempted to steady my breathing. I tried to relax. I closed my eyes. Then I opened them. Belatedly it occurred to me that I should inform my editors why I left the office four hours before my shift ended. I seemed to be operating in two realities. In the first, I was still mentally checking off tasks I had to complete. In the second, I was falling to pieces.

Still wrapped in my blanket, I sat down at my desk to email my editors. I noticed a new message from the *Globe*'s chief of security. He said he had forgotten to mention a second copy of the same death threat, also directed at me. It had gone straight to the executive offices because the envelope had been addressed to the publisher. Much later, I realized this meant the publisher likely knew about the threat to me, perhaps even before I did.

When the police cruiser pulled into my driveway, I shivered. I interviewed the police; they didn't interview me. The officer told me his name was Constable Mark White. Whenever I meet someone named White, I can't help blurting stupid puns.

So let's get this straight: you're White and I'm Wong.

This time I merely shook his hand, noting the red, white and blue "Toronto Police" patch on his sleeve. The officer was big and strong, or perhaps he was only average size, and he seemed big because I felt so frightened. He seemed sympathetic, too, certainly in comparison with the *Globe*'s security chief.

We sat down in my living room with Norman. The officer began taking notes, which calmed me down. He explained that he worked in the Major Crimes Unit at Fifty-Three Division, the precinct responsible for my neighborhood. He asked for a copy of my Dawson article. "Was your picture published with it?" he asked, scanning the front page. My feeling of calm evaporated. I pointed him to the inside page where my photo had indeed appeared. I knew it also was on the newspaper's website.

The killer knows what I look like.

Next Constable White studied the manila envelope. The postmark showed that it had been mailed two days earlier, at 1:06 P.M., from a post office in Montreal. The sender had gone to the trouble of attaching a blue airmail sticker and paying extra postage.

At this point, Norman walked over to my computer and began typing. A few moments later, he called over his shoulder, "I've got the post office." It was in Saint-Laurent, one of Montreal's largest neighborhoods.

"I think we can find the guy," Constable White said. "The post offices have video cameras, and the time stamp is on the envelope." He paused. "But no one should have touched the letter with bare hands."

"The head of security said it didn't matter," I said.

"Pardon me, miss," said Constable White, "but your head of security is an idiot."

He asked me to recount the events of the previous week. I mentioned the thousands of hate emails, the sawn-up books and the envelope containing either excrement or blood. Constable White asked where the last item was.

"The mail room threw it out," I said.

He sighed and closed his notebook. "You are in danger. Keep on all the lights around your house all night. Be alert when you leave the house."

I asked the police officer whether my husband and I should tell our sons. "That is up to you," he said.

Was my family in Montreal in danger?

"There is a risk that someone could throw a Molotov cocktail or firebomb them."

Constable White gave me my file number, 1812136. Then he shook hands with us and drove off. It was just 4 P.M. and school was just letting out across the street. Ben and Sam arrived home, saucer-eyed. They had seen the police cruiser in our driveway. Norman and I decided to tell the boys about the threat to explain why they must not to open the door to strangers or accept any packages.

"The police will protect us," I said, trying to sound confident.

The phone rang. It was a parent at the school who had seen the police cruiser and wanted to know if we were okay. I heard Sam, my thirteen-year-old, telling her about death threats and police protection. On top of everything else, I began worrying about whether other parents would let their children come over to play.

Norman said nothing after reading the threat, and I never asked. I didn't want to know. Now, several years later I feel strong enough to handle the details. "It was pretty nasty stuff," he says. "But I was not too concerned because I didn't actually believe the guy knew where you lived. I did not say that at the time because you were pretty upset. I thought that if I played down the threat a bit, it might have gotten you more upset. There definitely was a threat there and it should have been taken seriously."

That night I phoned my sister to warn her about Molotov cocktails. Norman called our backyard neighbor, a spirited lady in her eighties, who promised to keep an eye out for snipers. After everyone else went to sleep, I sat alone in our darkened living room. With the exterior lights blazing, I could see the backyard clearly. I thought I saw someone in the shrubbery, but I didn't move away from the window. I don't know why I didn't move.

What had I done to deserve this?

CHAPTER 5

The Working Wounded

I never had a bankable skill when I was growing up. In my first year at university, when an English professor asked what I planned to do for a living, I replied dreamily, "I want a job that is never boring."

"There is no such job," she said.

But I found one. As a reporter, I could go undercover into a Chinese opium den or underground into a Nova Scotia coal mine, investigate money laundering in Boston and write about prepubescent Olympic gymnasts in Atlanta. Or I could, as the muckraking Chicago journalist F.P. Dunne urged a century ago, "comfort the afflicted and afflict the comfortable."

I loved the art and craft of journalism. I thought about story ideas all the time. Journalism was my core, my identity. Was this a mistake?

For some people, work is a means to pay the rent. Others are so obsessed with work they might as well sleep at the office. At cocktail parties, we feel adrift until that essential question is answered: What do you do? We need to know so we can decide your worth and rank and, of course, whether we should waste another nanosecond talking to you. In a "Jobs-R-Us" culture, even children can't escape being judged by their ambition. As soon as toddlers can speak in whole sentences, we ask: What do you want to be when you grow up?

For twenty years I had lived and breathed the *Globe*. Each day I read it from cover to cover. Now the thought of it landing on my doorstep each morning nauseated me. For the first time in my life, I couldn't bear to read it or any other newspaper. After Constable White's visit, I wanted to cancel my subscription. I didn't even feel strong enough to call the *Globe*'s circulation department myself. Norman phoned for me.

This new helplessness surprised me. I had always been so tough. In 1989 as the People's Liberation Army shot its way into Tiananmen Square, I refused to be evacuated from Beijing. Later, I fought off a kidnapping attempt by plainclothes police. When the bureau car was stolen and I discovered the thieves were the Chinese police, I was eight-months months pregnant. I didn't hesitate to march down to the police station and make them give it back. (And then of course I wrote a story about it.)

Yet mental toughness, I would learn, is completely unrelated to depression. The strongest people have suffered severe, prolonged clinical depression—world leaders like Winston Churchill, Theodore Roosevelt and Menachem Begin; hard-nosed journalists like Mike Wallace of *60 Minutes* fame; soldiers like the Canadian general Romeo Dallaire; world-class athletes like tennis champion Monica Seles. Conversely, so-called weak people can sometimes tolerate pressures that devastate the strong. When the same terrifying events happen to a group of people, there is no common pattern of behavior. Some resist, some collapse and some become the walking wounded. Sometimes the very source of misery keeps a person going.

Holocaust survivors speak of being sustained by a life in opposition. Their resistance to the enemy kept them alive during the most traumatic moments. They would not commit suicide because they did not want to give satisfaction to their tormenters. But years later, after they are freed and there is no tyranny to oppose, the same survivors sometimes give up. In 1987, forty-two years after working as a slave laborer at Auschwitz, Primo Levi, the Italian chemist and writer, committed suicide. In his book, *The Drowned and the Saved*, he wrote about the sad, exhausting moment of leaving the concentration camp. "In the majority of cases, the hour of liberation was neither joyful nor lighthearted. For most it occurred against a background of destruction, slaughter, and suffering. Just as they felt they were again becoming men, that is, responsible, the sorrows of men returned; the sorrow of the dispersed or lost family; the universal suffering all around; their own exhaustion, which seemed definitive, past cure; the problems of a life to begin all over again amid the rubble, often alone."

Robert Sapolsky, a neurobiologist and author of *Why Zebras Don't Get Ulcers*, suggests that genes and possibly, in-utero development, influence how much trauma each individual can tolerate. He notes that in the face of undeniable stressors, some people do much better than others. Certainly no one, myself least of all, understood my vulnerability. At work only the librarian, the security office and management knew about the death threat. Of course, my co-workers had seen the criticism of me in our newspaper and other media, but they probably assumed I was fine. After all, I was supposed to be one of the toughest reporters in the newsroom. I once had tremendous tolerance for stress. I assumed my resilience was limitless.

But I had never before been the target of racial attacks, an Internet stoning and public criticism in the media, including my own newspaper. I had never before been investigated by management, ordered not to speak or accused of disobeying a management order, and certainly not all of the above at once. One death threat earlier in my career had left me unscathed. Now, another pushed me over the edge. I had reached my personal flipping-out point. My deep emotional investment in my work set me up for a major depressive episode.

I work, therefore I am. Without my job, I didn't know who I was. I had always willingly put in long hours, about two or three hundred extra hours a year judging by the overtime on my pay slips. And I wasn't alone. Since 1967, Americans have averaged an extra 160 hours a year, equivalent to an additional month at the office. Canadians, measured by a combination of employment rate and total hours worked, rank fourth among the world's workaholics after Iceland in first place, New Zealand and Switzerland tied for second and Denmark in third.

Our culture holds that work is good. Therefore, not working makes us feel guilty. More and more people are working nights and weekends and even during vacations, especially since the advent of the Internet, the BlackBerry and the iPhone. Yet two longitudinal studies in the United States show that men who regularly take holidays are 32 percent less likely to die from a heart attack than those who keep working. Women who take vacations halve their risk. Even so, many employees can't or won't take time off. In Canada, only three out of four workers take all the vacation time they're owed, despite getting just nineteen days a year, less vacation time than almost any other country. The only developed nations with fewer are the Japanese (fifteen days) and the Americans (thirteen days).

Competition, debt and insecurity push people to work even harder during a recession. Unfortunately, this creates a vicious cycle for your mental health. If you keep working nights and weekends—and the sharp decline in leisure time shows that many are—you have no time to bowl, volunteer at your church, play guitar or otherwise develop a healthier identity independent of your job. But over-identification with work can lead to anxiety, panic attacks, post-traumatic stress disorder (PTSD) and depression.

The International Labor Organization of the United Nations now calls occupational stress a global epidemic. Many of life's most stressful events involve the workplace—firings, layoffs, performance reviews, tension among team members, increased responsibility, longer hours and, of course, trouble with the boss. Workers joke about taking "mental-health days," but it's no laughing matter: three out of four American workers report that theirs is a stressful workplace. And in the United States, 60 percent of lost workdays each year are stress-related. In a survey reported in *The Wall Street Journal*, one-third of employees considered quitting because of stress and 14 percent actually quit. In Canada, mental illness accounts for 40 percent of all disability claims and sick leaves. Stress-related expenses include ballooning absenteeism, lower productivity, higher staff turnover, increased workers' compensation and costlier medical insurance.

Workplace stress triggered my depression, but I did not understand that at first. Initially I didn't even accept that I had depression. I thought I merely needed time to recharge. I didn't yet know there are two kinds of depression. One type occurs without external triggers and is caused by predisposing factors such as heredity. The other type is caused by a crisis—a job loss or a death in the family. Some experts would say that it's distorting to separate the two types because many people who suffer from depression have a combination of an internal predisposition and an external trigger.

In fact, both types of depression have the same impact on the body. Both shrink the brain's hippocampus, the seahorse-shaped gateway through which all new emotional memories must pass. (Post-traumatic stress disorder causes a similar shrinkage in the hippocampus. Confusingly, PTSD can masquerade as depression or bipolar disorder and symptoms can arise later on, far from the battlefield or the original stressors.)

Both types of depression are chemically identical and both have a wide-ranging impact affecting:

- neurotransmitter function
- synaptic function
- increased or decreased excitability between neurons
- alteration of gene expression
- hypometabolism or hypermetabolism in the frontal cortex
- heightened levels of thyroid-releasing hormone (TRH)
- disrupted function of the amygdala (crucial for computing the emotional significance of events)
- increased or decreased levels of melatonin (the hormone important in regulating the circadian rhythms of several biological functions)
- increased prolactin (a hormone of the pituitary gland)
- less fluctuation of circadian body temperature
- malfunction of the circuit linking the thalamus, basal ganglia and frontal lobes (which control working-memory activities)
- increased blood flow to the frontal lobe; decreased flow to the occipital lobe

Scientists aren't sure which of the above changes *cause* depression and which are merely the brain's way of *fighting* depression. Two key changes, however, always occur with the onset of depression. There is an increased level of cortisol, a "fight-or-flight" hormone secreted by the adrenal gland, and a decreased level of serotonin, a hormone that acts as a neurotransmitter in the brain.

Unlike cortisol, which can be calibrated indirectly through urine, serotonin levels can't be measured. Consequently, there is currently no chemical test for depression. Nor is there scientific evidence that depressed people experience an "imbalance" of serotonin. Doctors only know that serotonin seems to cushion the effects of the illness. And they know that serotonin-enhancing drugs can initiate a process that helps depressed people gradually to improve their mood.

Intriguingly, scientists have recently noted a correlation between depression and smoking. About 40 to 50 percent of people diagnosed with depression are smokers, more than double the 20 percent of smokers in the general population. As nicotine appears to have the same effect as antidepressants on brain activity and mood, smoking may in fact be a subconscious attempt to self-medicate the symptoms of depression. Researchers such as Dr. Verner Knott, a scientist at the University of Ottawa and the Royal Ottawa Mental Health Centre, are trying to develop new treatments for depression that mimic the effects of nicotine without the health risk of smoking.

There is no typical depression. Major depression can be so disabling you cannot work. Yet some individuals react to depression by working even harder. Charles Darwin frequently complained of "fits," "air fatigues," "hysterical crying" and "head symptoms" that left him "not able to do anything one day out of three." Yet the pain of his depression may have provided the excuse to withdraw from everything superfluous to concentrate on his research. His work was his "sole enjoyment in life," a welcome escape from his gloom. "Work is the only thing which makes life endurable to me," Darwin wrote, according to Jonah Lehrer, author of How We Decide.

In the midst of my depression, a retired journalist in Toronto invited me for coffee and volunteered her own experience. Her own depression had been severe and had lasted more than a year. Yet she had continued filing five newspaper columns a week while raising three young children and supporting her husband's budding political career. No one had any inkling she was sick, not even her husband. With antidepressants and a prolonged spa vacation, she eventually recovered. Now, years later, the only tangible evidence of that hard year was her decaying teeth. The meds had given her dry mouth and the lack of saliva had ruined her enamel.

I couldn't work at all. After Dawson, every piece of hate email, every attack on my family, every perceived betrayal by my newspaper chipped away at my brimming self-confidence. No one expected this consequence, least of all myself. I had been infamous for skewering celebrities over lunch and then writing up the encounter. "The Hannibal Lecter of the lunch set," one victim complained. The "Queen of Mean," a rival journalist grumped. I never thought I was mean. I worked the celebrity beat like any other, did my research, observed and asked hard questions. Four out of five got a positive write-up. (Yes, I counted.) But I admit I dished it out. And I thought I could take it, too. I wasn't thin-skinned. Or was I?

The psyche is exquisitely fragile. And the Dawson attacks seemed different from previous criticism. For the first time people attacked my gender. They told me to go back to China. They said I was ugly and had slanted eyes. Other media had piled on, calling me "stupid," "misguided" and a "disgrace to journalism." Even so, I believe I could have withstood those attacks if only someone in management had offered one word of support. But when my company wouldn't even call the police for me, the betrayal felt absolute. I had been pilloried, reviled, savaged and threatened with death, yet my workplace seemed unwilling to protect me. Everything unraveled.

A psychological emergency is invisible. Major depression invades your body, replacing your former self with a paler, ghost-like version. There's no bruising or bleeding. You cannot see the wounds. Even I did not understand the urgency of getting treatment. I only knew that I felt hopeless and was weeping all the time. By the end of the second week of unrelenting attacks, I felt a desperate need to see my family doctor. I didn't think I was actually sick, but I didn't know what else to do. I phoned for an appointment but couldn't get through. Uncharacteristically, I gave up.

Instead, I went downtown for the memorial service for Ken Thomson, the owner of *The Globe and Mail*. He had died of a heart attack a few months earlier at the age of eighty-three. Thomson had been the richest man in Canada and the ninth richest person in the world. I liked him anyway. A hereditary British peer, he eschewed the title and shopped for his own groceries, walked his own dogs and made his son drive him to the airport. As a volunteer for the Toronto Humane Society, he also walked abandoned dogs. He was preternaturally shy, but always friendly. After I returned from my six-year posting in Beijing, he occasionally phoned me or sent a note. When I spoke at the Toronto Hunt club, where he was a member, he came to the dinner, but declined the organizers' invitation to sit at the head table.

Despite my state of mind, I was determined to pay tribute to Thomson.

He had been an exemplary newspaper proprietor, astute enough to keep his hands off the newsroom and generous enough to provide the money to let reporters do their job. At the memorial service at Roy Thomson Hall, the iconic, funnel-shaped symphony hall named for his father, I took a seat in the balcony. The family had flown in Men of the Deeps, a choir of coal miners from Cape Breton Island, Nova Scotia. As they marched into the darkened hall, illuminated only by the lights on their miner's helmets, their voices filled the space. Then Joaquin Valdepeñas, principal clarinetist of the Toronto Symphony Orchestra, played the *Adagio* from Mozart's Clarinet Concerto in A Major. For the first time in my life, music moved me to tears. I wept for the passing of a man, for journalism and for myself. Suddenly I missed Ken Thomson terribly.

Although the memorial service calmed me somewhat, I still felt desperate as I left the concert hall. Stepping out in the autumn sun, I realized my doctor's office was just a few blocks away. Perhaps if I just showed up she might squeeze me in. I walked over and took an elevator to the second floor. As usual, her receptionist was behind a high counter, shielded by a thick plate-glass window.

"I need to see Dr. Au," I whispered. For some reason I didn't want the other patients in the waiting room to hear.

"We're fully booked for today," the receptionist snapped. "She can see you next month."

"I need to see her *today*," I begged softly.

"What's wrong?" The receptionist's shrill voice bounced off the glass.

I cringed. By now I was sure the other patients had pricked up their ears. What *was* wrong with me? I wasn't bleeding. I wasn't limping. I didn't even have a low-grade fever.

"I'm not sleeping," I croaked. It sounded lame, but I didn't know what else to say. I certainly didn't want her or anyone else to know I was crying all the time. To my embarrassment, my eyes filled with tears.

"The earliest I can book you is next Tuesday at 6:30 P.M."

That was five days away, an eternity. I didn't feel I could hang on that long, but I had no choice. I nodded silently and skulked away.

Two years later, I dropped by my doctor's office for a routine appointment. I was no longer severely depressed. Indeed, I had started writing again and, a few days earlier, had written the above paragraphs about that desperate moment. To my surprise, much had changed since then. The counter was no longer so high. The glass barrier wasn't very thick, either. The receptionist, the same person, did not sound shrill. I listened carefully as she spoke to a patient on the telephone. She wasn't brusque, just businesslike.

"There are no facts, only interpretations," the German philosopher, Nietzsche, famously observed. So how to account for the discrepancy in my perception? Looking back, I must have reached a saturation point for emotional abuse. I had become hypersensitive, the way even a gentle touch on a broken ankle hurts like hell. In my wounded state, everything had become magnified: the volume of the receptionist's voice, the height of the counter, the thickness of the glass. It wasn't objective reality, but it was *my* reality.

Back at my office, I could hardly wait for the workday, and the workweek, to end. It was a Friday. Normally, I would race the clock all week, trying to squeeze in an extra rewrite, a bit more reporting. I would always be shocked at how fast Friday arrived. But now, two weeks after my Dawson story was published, I couldn't bear to stay a minute longer in Toronto.

By chance, four friends and I had planned a girls' weekend at a cottage on Lake Erie. Right after work that afternoon, we escaped in my van. Luckily one of them offered to drive because I immediately began recounting everything that had happened, including the death threat. I talked and cried, and cried and talked, for the entire five-hour drive—six, if you include the hour when we stopped for pizza and a glass of wine and, yes, I kept talking.

When we arrived at the highway restaurant for dinner, I was mortified to discover my period had started and my khaki shorts were stained with blood. One friend, Brenda, pressed herself behind me and escorted me, in lockstep, into the washroom. For a moment, the others thought that the gunman had found me and Brenda was trying to protect me. They rushed after us into the ladies' room, where we all dissolved into hysterical laughter. While the others ordered dinner, Brenda passed me wet paper towels and went out to the van to fetch Tampax and clean clothes. When we finally sat down at the table, everyone started laughing again. I joined in and couldn't stop. All I needed, it seemed, were some friends to listen to me.

Women instinctively know that talking to friends is therapeutic. In fact, talking to almost anyone helps as long as your listener is intelligent and insightful. A famous 1979 study found that English professors with both these qualities were as able as trained therapists to help psychiatric patients. My mother, Eva, experienced this therapeutic effect when she became briefly suicidal after getting married, giving up nursing and having four children in six years. She poured out her woes to her family doctor. "I was fine after that," Mom told me years later. "I felt much better."

Talking about your misery actually changes brain activity for the better.

In fact, researchers have found talk therapy as effective as antidepressant drugs. A landmark Toronto study of patients who had recovered from depression found that both cognitive behavioral therapy and drug therapy caused definitive changes in brain imaging. "It's just tapping into a different component of the same depression circuit board," Helen Mayberg, a neuroscientist at the University of Texas at San Antonio, wrote in the 2004 study.

My cellphone rang as my friends and I were climbing back into the van after dinner. It was the police. A detective informed me that the fingerprint lab was working on the death-threat letter. He added that my home address was now tagged in the 911 computers. "Any calls for service get an immediate notification of the threat situation, so the response will be speeded up."

Back in the van I started shivering again. For the rest of our road trip, several more hours, I talked nonstop while my poor friends sighed and nodded in sympathy. Finally we arrived at the cottage. It was nearly midnight. Although it was late September, the pool had been cranked up to near-tropical temperature. We all plunged in. Floating silently under the stars, in saltwater as warm as amniotic fluid, I stopped obsessing about editors, publishers and death threats. Far from Toronto, I suddenly felt safe. That night I fell asleep to the sound of waves lapping at the shore. For the first time in two weeks, I slept deeply.

When I woke up on Saturday, it was nearly noon. Liz was back from a run. Cara was making mashed potatoes. Brenda was drinking coffee. Rosabel was reading a glossy magazine. I sat down in the kitchen in my nightgown and nibbled on a slice of delicious homemade banana bread. "You can't go into work on Monday," said Liz, as she poured me a cup of coffee.

"You're not in any shape to go to the office," Cara agreed.

"You need some time off," Brenda said.

"You have to call in sick and then see what your doctor says," said Liz.

But how could I be *sick*? I had just slept for twelve glorious hours. Whatever was bothering me seemed to have vanished. I was looking forward to another swim, a hike through the nearby wetlands, some window-shopping and a chick flick on the DVD-player.

Suddenly I heard footsteps on the porch. A man was speaking English with a French-Canadian accent. I suppressed a scream.

The gunman has found me.

If I had had a gun, I would have shot first and asked questions later. But it was only Remi, Liz's next-door neighbor and handyman, dropping by to discuss some renovations. The French-Canadian accent had never had that effect on me before. As a Montrealer, it had once symbolized home to me, a madeleine-like remembrance of summer jobs, of working at a fast-food counter where I pumped paper cups of cold Pepsi and spoke high-school French to customers. Now, hearing the same accent sparked Pavlovian panic. My hair-trigger reaction surprised me.

Perhaps I do need a few days off.

The rest of the weekend was restorative. We barbecued steaks and ate Cara's delicious mashed potatoes, oozing milk, butter and cheese. We swam in the obscenely warm pool. We shopped for pashminas at Dollarama. We sunned ourselves in Liz's backyard, with its landscaped dunes and expansive view of Lake Erie. On Sunday, I slept again until noon. I had trouble opening my eyes. My bones felt like liquid. I could hardly get out of bed. After so many sleepless nights, I assumed that slumbering until midday was a good sign. I thought it meant I was getting better.

I am okay. I can go into work tomorrow.

That night, after a blissful, healing weekend with my friends, I returned to Toronto, dropped everyone off and drove home in my van. Then I spotted the gunman's pickup truck across the street and fell apart.

CHAPTER 6

Crack-Up

The therapeutic effects of the cottage weekend vaporized in a flash. Back home, I was terrified anew of a sniper taking me out. Outside the house, sidewalk newspaper boxes tormented me, reminding me of the poisonous emails, security's refusal to call the police, the publisher's investigation. I cried incessantly.

"Too much anger and too many tears. At three o'clock in the morning, a forgotten package has the same tragic importance as a death sentence," F. Scott Fitzgerald wrote in *The Crack-Up*, his three-part series on his own breakdown published in *Esquire* magazine in 1936.

Taking my friends' advice, I called in sick that Monday and Tuesday, counting down the hours until my evening appointment with my family doctor. I arrived half an hour early. To my relief, the receptionist had already left for the day. It wasn't just her strident voice and brusque manner (as I then perceived it). I also felt an inchoate sense of shame about being there merely for crying. The journalist in me did note that I had never minded in the past when the same receptionist handed me a plastic container for a urine sample. So why did I suddenly feel embarrassed now? It seems that I sensed the stigma, even before I understood that I was suffering a mental collapse.

My doctor came out to the waiting room in her usual white lab coat. Susan Au, a Chinese-Canadian in her fifties, has short salt-and-pepper hair and glasses that sometimes slip down her nose. I had become her patient nearly twenty years earlier when I moved to Toronto and had instantly liked her. She is serious and sincere, a conservative, meticulous doctor who during annual physicals even inspects the soles of my feet for cancerous moles. She never rushes me through an appointment, and always takes the time to answer questions.

Dr. Au ushered me into her tiny office, closed the door and asked me what was wrong. Normally, I see her once a year, if that. This time I burst into tears. Through deep, wracking sobs, I gave her the condensed cottage-route version. It still took almost forty-five minutes to recount. When I finished, she said quietly, "I think you need two weeks off."

I felt a load lift from my shoulders. *Two whole weeks will save my life.* At the same time, I felt a spasm of grief. *Two weeks means I'm a lot worse than I thought.* I wasn't recovering from open-heart surgery. Sure, I couldn't sleep, I couldn't read and the very thought of being in the newsroom plunged me into despair. But I could walk and talk. I wasn't wearing my shirt inside out. Surely I could just snap out of it?

As the tears coursed down my face, Dr. Au scribbled a note. "You need to rest," she said, writing me my first-ever sick note. "The employer doesn't need to know anything except that you are sick. That's the law."

She handed me the note. I glanced at it: "I certify that the above named was absent from work October 4 until October 23, 2006, for medical reasons."

Next she wrote out two prescriptions, one for Imovane and one for Ativan. Over the years I had taken Imovane, a sleeping pill, sparingly, usually half a pill at a time, whenever deadline pressures kept me awake. Because Imovane was addictive, Dr. Au had always limited me to ten pills a year. Now she gave me a prescription for thirty pills. Ativan, Dr. Au said, was a tranquilizer. "Take it when you're feeling anxious. You don't swallow it. You put it under your tongue."

I told my doctor that I didn't think I could lie in bed for two weeks with pills under my tongue.

"Don't stay in bed," she said, smiling for the first time. "Go for walks. Go to the movies. You like music—go to the symphony. Do some gardening. Try to get out of town. Travel. It would be really good if you could get away."

"How can I go on vacation if I'm supposed to be sick?"

"You are under a lot of stress at work. This is the best cure."

Dr. Au herself had been at work for nearly eleven hours. I knew I had overstayed my appointment. On the street, clutching my sick note and the two prescriptions, I started crying again. It was rush hour. No one gave me a second glance, a benefit of living in a city of four million strangers. I went to the nearest pharmacy and had the prescriptions filled.

On the subway home, I considered Dr. Au's advice. Two weeks off, with pay, to have a good time going to concerts, felt faintly fraudulent. And travel. How could I call in sick *and* then go on vacation? Could she be right that the cure for crying was gardening and gallivanting? What kind of illness was this?

At home, I told my family about Dr. Au's miraculous cure. A day later, Ben said, "I've got tickets to the symphony." I bit my tongue to avoid blurting out: "But you hate classical concerts!" Instead, I swiftly accepted the offer before he changed his mind. Only later it dawned on me that my sixteen-year-old had taken the doctor's advice to heart and had decided to help his mom get well. At the time, I was so mired in misery that I had failed to grasp the most touching and thoughtful of gestures.

That Saturday evening, the Toronto Symphony Orchestra played the *Adagietto* from Mahler's Symphony No. 5. To my surprise, the doleful descending passages felt like a balm. To my further surprise, research has found that misery does love company, that melancholy songs comfort sad people by signaling that they are not alone. Conversely, happy music—those damn Christmas songs piped through a shopping-mall sound system—does not cheer up sad people. Instead it irritates them and makes them feel isolated, as if no one understands them.

Next a Norwegian pianist, Leif Ove Andsnes, played Beethoven's Piano Concerto No. 3 in C Minor. I lost myself in the first movement, a muscular and emotionally turbulent *Allegro con brio*. During the *Largo* that followed, the music grew soft and Ben, whose tastes ran more to folk-rock groups like Great Lake Swimmers, fell sound asleep. At intermission, I revived him with a chocolate-almond ice-cream bar. He managed to stay awake for the final piece, Beethoven's Symphony No. 7 in A Major.

The evening with my son was magical. Then I went home, switched on the radio and heard that unknown assailants had shot to death a Russian investigative journalist. Anna Politkovskaya had angered authorities by probing into Russian atrocities in Chechnya. Her murder half a world away deepened my own sense of vulnerability. I was still afraid to turn on the lights in my living room. Periodically I checked the backyard for assassins, as the journalist in me sourly noted that, on top of everything else, I now had to worry about someone shooting out my recently installed, low E-coated, argon-gas-filled, double-glazed, thermal windows.

Although I took the sleeping pills Dr. Au had prescribed, I routinely awoke at 3 A.M., feeling exhausted and unable to fall back asleep. Depression was the cause of my insomnia, but insomnia deepened my depression. Imovane left a bitter taste at the back of my throat. I began having an upset stomach and diarrhea. My memory frayed. I couldn't recall conversations, tasks or simple facts. I feared answering the phone. When friends left messages of concern, I couldn't muster the energy to call them back, which depressed me further.

I filled the prescription for Ativan, but was afraid to take them. Even in my distressed state, it struck me as tragicomic that anti-anxiety pills were making me anxious. Also known by the generic name, lorazepam, Ativan is addictive. The night Michael Jackson died of heart failure, his physician had given him several injections of liquid Ativan. The drug is a benzodiazepine, a class of psychoactive tranquilizers that slow the central nervous system. In 1963 "benzos" famously hit the market under the brand name Valium. Tranquilizers do not, by themselves, alleviate depression. In fact, they can actually *make* you depressed over the long-term. Their magic is in providing instant (albeit temporary) relief from anxiety. Recreationally, benzos are used as a means of "coming down" from amphetamine-induced highs from speed or Ecstasy.

I faxed my sick note to the human-resources department. The vice-president emailed back within an hour saying she had received only my cover letter. For the next four days, I faxed and re-faxed Dr. Au's note. Each time my fax machine confirmed a successful transmission. And each time, the HR department told me it had received only my cover letter, not the actual doctor's note.

What on earth was going on? I became hysterical about my sick note. I felt that unless it arrived in the HR office, I was AWOL. Depression and anxiety are the chicken-and-egg conundrum of mental illness. Too much anxiety can lead to depression, but depression fuels anxiety. The ostensible failure of my fax to go through took on "the same tragic importance as a death sentence," that Fitzgerald described. Looking back, my old journalistic self would have solved the problem in seconds. I could have scanned the sick note and emailed it. I could have sent it by courier or snail mail. I could even have taken it in upon my return. Surely the *Globe* would not mind considering that, in twenty years, I had taken a total of two or three sick days. But the old, competent me had vanished. I stood anxiously beside the fax machine in Norman's study, crying and wringing my hands.

"What am I going to do?" I wailed.

"I'll *drive* it down."

I stopped in mid-wail. "You will?"

Normally, my husband gets cranky when I ask him to run errands. In fact, on such occasions he often suffers from temporary spousal deafness syndrome so that I have to repeat myself. (Of course, when I don't want him to hear something, he can hear me fine from the far side of the house.)

On the Saturday of Thanksgiving weekend, Norman drove the one-hour round trip to the *Globe* to drop off my sick note. When he returned, I was still on edge.

"Did you deliver it?"

"Yes," he said patiently.

"Who did you hand it to?" I demanded.

"The security guard at the front desk."

I exhaled. I had been a damsel in distress, and Norman had ridden to my rescue. What a guy.

Two days later, a courier rang my doorbell and handed me an envelope. Inside was a blurred, much-photocopied authorization form. By signing it, I would be authorizing an "intervention specialist" at Manulife Financial to talk to anyone at all who knew anything private about me. Specifically, it said: "any person or organization with personal information." Even in my fog of despair, I noticed that the form had no expiration date. If I signed it, the authorization would be permanent.

In a separate note, the *Globe*'s human resources department instructed me to sign the form within forty-eight hours or forfeit all my sick pay and benefits. I had been sick only a few days. Did my employer not believe my doctor's note? Why the threat to cut off my benefits and pay? And why was a complete stranger, someone who didn't even work for my company, empowered to talk to others about me?

Not understanding why something bad is happening increases a sense of powerlessness, which in turn deepens depression. Yet at my core I remained the same tough person I was before I fell sick. It turned out that my company had recently outsourced management of short-term sick leave to Manulife. A friend told me a typical authorization form restricts disclosure to relevant *medical* information from *medical* personnel. The *Globe*'s expansive form would let Manulife talk to anyone it wanted, including all my ex-husbands (if I had any). I had nothing to hide, but I saw no reason to relinquish my right to privacy. I crossed out "any person or organization," wrote in Dr. Au's name and phone number, signed the form and faxed it back.

I asked my union rep about the authorization form. (Yes, I was a union member, part of the Communications, Energy and Paperworkers Union of Canada, Local 87-M, that represented everyone from journalists to sawmill workers.) My rep advised against signing the form and said the union would file a grievance against the *Globe*. It turned out that the newspaper had introduced the form six months earlier without notifying the union, a violation of the collective agreement.

Thus did I unwittingly ignite a battle royal over a *form*. The hostilities would draw in the *Globe*'s parent company, Bell Canada Enterprises, one of Canada's biggest companies, which had recently imposed the new form on all 54,000 of its employees. It would also embroil Manulife, Canada's biggest insurance company, which had drawn up the form. And soon I, too, would become ensnared in a Catch-22 of disability and sick pay because, in the end, it wasn't about health. It was about money.

According to the collective agreement, *Globe* employees who fell ill were entitled to full pay and benefits in the short term, defined as six months. The *Globe*, like many companies, paid short-term disability to employees out of its own coffers. Some time earlier, however, the *Globe* had hired a third party to *adjudicate* its short-term sick claims. That third party was Manulife. If Manulife agreed that you were sick, the *Globe* would issue short-term sick pay. But if Manulife said you weren't sick, you would be ordered back to work and, of course, you wouldn't get sick pay.

Then it gets interesting. According to the contract, short-term disability was the pre-condition for any claim for long-term disability payments. So unless Manulife agreed that you were sick in the short term, you had no hope of moving on to long-term disability, a generous and significant amount that just happened to be paid by ... Manulife.

The grievance and the battle royal and my understanding of Manulife's conflicting roles would all come later. At the beginning, I only knew I would not relinquish my privacy rights. That day, as I studied the blurred photocopied form and the ultimatum from human resources, I began to weep. I fumbled for my orange plastic cylinder of Ativan pills, twisted open the childproof top and shook one out. The pill was powder blue, round and smaller than a peppercorn. I wedged it under my tongue where it melted into a grainy slush. My pulse slowed. Tears still ran down my cheeks, but I stopped sobbing. It was my first tranquilizer and I loved it.

When I calmed down, I returned a call from the HR vice-president. She answered on the second ring. She assured me the form was standard procedure and that there was no hidden agenda. She also urged me to talk to the Manulife intervention specialist. "She's a very lovely lady. Manulife wants to make sure you're getting the right treatment."

Then the HR vice-president suddenly switched topics. Had I spoken to a *National Post* columnist named Andrew Coyne? I was confused and said I had not. I had no idea what she was talking about. She said that Coyne had written about the attacks on me.

"We think you caused the column," the HR vice-president said.

I burst into tears. I explained that I had stopped reading all newspapers two weeks earlier. I told her that I had obeyed the management directive not to talk to the media. I had not spoken to the columnist and had no intention of doing so.

Looking back, it seems surreal. I was the one who was mentally ill, yet the company was acting paranoid. I felt another panic attack coming on. After the call ended, I dissolved into heaving sobs. Norman stood by helplessly. The muscle under my left eye began twitching. I slipped another Ativan under my tongue. The crying stopped.

PART II

DENIAL

CHAPTER 7

The Geographic Cure

I am lurking outside the Culinary Institute of America (CIA) in Hyde Park, New York. It's lunchtime. My heart is pounding, but in a good way. I feel alive again. As a journalist, I always thrived on going where I wasn't wanted. Now I'm about to carry out a covert operation inside the CIA itself. I'm going to break the code, the dress code, that is, at Escoffier, one of four student-staffed restaurants. The dining room bans jeans and sneakers, which, alas, are what I'm wearing.

Gigi and my cousin-in-law, Colleen, are properly attired and have already snagged a table. I'll wait until the maitre d' steps away.

There he goes.

I dash across the room and dive into a chair. Draping the snowy tablecloth around my hips, I order a sampler of soups—oxtail, lemongrass and cream of mushroom, followed by arugula salad and a seared medallion of beef atop a purée of potato and roasted garlic. My companions beam; apparently I haven't been eating much.

A few days earlier, my sister had expressed a desire to visit upstate New York. By what seemed a strange coincidence, Dad and Colleen wanted to come, too. Just as I had missed the thoughtfulness of my son's invitation to the concert, I didn't understand that they, too, had taken Dr. Au's recommendations to heart. In fact, upstate New York was the last place Dad, who had difficulty walking more than five minutes, would want to spend a weekend. His tastes ran to cigars and football games, not the rococo mansions of the Gilded Age. Personally, I adored rococo. What's more, fleeing Toronto meant escaping the seemingly incessant phone calls, emails and couriered letters from work. I had reached the point where I was so agitated I was asking Colleen to return calls from the Manulife intervention specialist.

Stress activates the body's primitive fight-or-flight mechanism, and I was in flight mode. My adrenal glands were spewing adrenalin, cortisol and other hormones into my system, tensing muscles, constricting blood vessels, quickening my pulse and slowing my digestive tract. As my train glided out of Union Station in Toronto, I felt my shoulders relax. I stopped clenching my jaw. It seemed as if an iron vise had been removed from my head. Dr. Au was right. Getting away was a huge relief.

As I gazed at the sparkling expanse of Lake Ontario, framed by leaves of gold and scarlet, I was glad I had splurged on a first-class ticket. Normally I see no compelling reason to pay anything but the cheapest fare, but the free-for-all system in economy class suddenly posed an insurmountable challenge. In first class I was guaranteed a reserved seat. In my hypersensitive state, I could not cope with the clenched smiles elicited by asking, "Is this seat taken?" I could not bear spending the trip beside someone unfriendly, at least, as I perceived it. William Styron, the American writer, described a similar feeling of inadequacy in *Darkness Visible*, his memoir of depression:

> *Of the many dreadful manifestations of the disease, both physical and psychological, a sense of self-hatred—or, put less categorically, a failure of self-esteem—is one of the most universally experienced symptoms, and I had suffered more and more from a general feeling of worthlessness as the malady had progressed.*

I got off the train in Cornwall, Ontario. Colleen happened to be working there at the time, and the next day we drove an hour further east to Montreal to pick up Dad and Gigi. I tensed as we approached the city limits. This was my thought: my would-be assassin lives here. And though it seems ludicrous now, I half-expected people to be lined up along the road, hurling insults at me. The streets were, of course, quite normal.

To my relief, my father and sister were waiting by the door. We left immediately for the U.S. border. We apparently were a suspicious combination: an elderly Chinese man, two middle-aged Chinese women and a blue-eyed blonde claiming to be a relative. The U.S. border guard quizzed us on our family structure and then asked where we were headed.

"Hyde Park," Gigi replied.

"What's there?" he asked, mystified.

"The birthplace of Roosevelt."

He shook his head and waved us through.

"I should have told them I was your father's trophy wife but that he couldn't afford much," Colleen said. Dad laughed so hard, she added, "Bill, if you don't quit laughing, I'll be insulted." Dad laughed harder. Colleen laughed, too, and my sister and I joined in. I had crossed the border. I felt safe.

In Hyde Park, Dad stayed close by the hotel watching football on television while the rest of us toured Springwood, the palatial family estate of Franklin Delano Roosevelt. Later we visited the six-hundred-acre Vanderbilt estate, owned by the richest robber baron of all time. Built with a fortune amassed before the nuisance of personal income tax, the nineteenth-century mansion had its own stables, docks, railway station and hydroelectric plant. The third floor alone had thirteen bedrooms to house the personal maids that accompanied each guest. The gilded dining room boasted sweeping views of the Hudson River. We gawked at the mahogany table, set for thirty guests for a pink-themed luncheon: pink china, pink flowers, pink crystal wineglasses and an all-pink menu from soup to fish to dessert.

Just as my weekend at Liz's cottage had been therapeutic, traipsing through an all-pink dining room was a balm. I began to understand what the novelist Elizabeth McCracken in her memoir, *An Exact Replica of a Figment of My Imagination*, called the geographic cure. After her first child was stillborn, she dealt with her grief by traveling incessantly, up bell towers and monuments, to deserted beaches and quiet restaurants. It helped immensely. Yet she also notes, "You can't out-travel sadness. You will find it has smuggled itself along in your suitcase."

Although the sadness stayed with me, travel did transport me away from the rancid crust of everyday misery. When I stayed in Toronto unexpected triggers kept sending little poisoned darts into my heart. The radio broadcast stories about Quebec's treatment of immigrants. Newspaper boxes loomed like Venus flytraps. And why were so many buildings in Toronto labeled "Manulife"? Here in upstate New York, I could walk safely down the street. I could lose myself in the Gilded Age.

When Dr. Au first prescribed trips out of town, it seemed too much like playing hooky. My notion of illness was firmly rooted in the physical. To me, sick meant a fever, vomiting and the like, for which the treatment included lying in bed in a darkened room. I could not conceive of an illness for which the cure was indistinguishable from a vacation. Having tried it, however, I now know that my doctor was right.

Fleeing the stressor helps. It is why, when lovers fight, one side invariably storms out. It's why, when a teenager rebels, she moves out (and the parents are so thrilled they want to break open a bottle of Champagne). The geographic cure enables you to go where no one knows you, where you don't have to talk about yourself or your problems, where conversations are gratifyingly superficial, where the most challenging question you are likely to be asked is: where are you from?

Travel means being distracted by new details, new things, new logistics. How do you get from the airport to your hotel? Where is that museum, that bistro, that boutique? How do you operate the television remote? You can sit at a sidewalk café all day observing others, looking like you're part of the action, but no one forces you to participate. You can partake of life safely from the sidelines.

Once you check into your hotel, you are anonymous, a sixteen-digit number on a credit card (although the better ones will attempt a false intimacy by addressing you by name, read off that same credit card). At 4 A.M., when you can't sleep, you can go out and explore a new city. Or you can lie in bed all day. No one is there to urge you to get up and at 'em. Hotels are blissfully infantilizing, with someone else making your bed, just like when you were a child. In a good hotel, you can even get turndown service with a chocolate truffle on the pillow—the adult version of being tucked in at night. You can shut out the whole world by hanging a sign on your doorknob. If only I could have worn a do-not-disturb sign at work.

In Michael Cunningham's novel *The Hours*, a depressed housewife in Los Angeles checks herself into a hotel just so she can read Virginia Woolf for a few undisturbed hours and then, perhaps, kill herself. "This hotel, this lobby, is precisely what she wants—the cool nowhere of it, the immaculate non-smell, the brisk unemotional comings and goings."

That's what I longed for, too.

According to Dr. Au, the geographic cure was not confined to traveling the earth, but could be extended to include digging and planting in it, too. I was skeptical about her recommendation of gardening. How would sticking things in dirt help me? Wasn't this just a cliché—planting, growing, blossoming, renewal?

I am not a gardener. I love gardens—the way Marie Antoinette loved Versailles. When we renovated our house a few years earlier, I asked the architect to design an L-shaped flowerbed along the driveway. I envisioned my own small corner of Versailles, with beds of tea roses and manicured boxwood. That first spring I prevailed upon Norman and Ben, then ten years old, to dig out the hard, stony clay and replace it with a truckload of topsoil, loam and peat moss. Next I planted dozens of hot-pink and magenta impatiens, a miracle flower that blooms in the shade. The seedlings came tightly encased in plastic four-packs. Too tightly. When I tried to extract the seedlings, I usually ripped off half their roots. I also planted peonies, tulips and some perennials whose names I can't remember, mainly because they are no longer with us. Who knew you had to water flowers? And a related question: how come weeds flourish without water?

As the years passed and the weeds won, I gave up. Now, on the advice of my doctor, I was willing to try again. Costco.com offered a five-hundred-bulb deal, with a choice of a purple-pink set or a red-yellow set. I preferred the girly purple-pink combo, but made the mistake of asking Norman and the boys for their preference. It was another sign of how far I had fallen. Until Dawson, I had always made up my own mind on all matters not involving hockey gear or power tools. And in the past, whenever I had taken a family vote, I behaved like a permanent member of the UN Security Council. Everyone had a vote, but I had the veto.

Norman professed to have no clear opinion on bulb colors, although he may merely have been striving for emotional distance from any further relationship with the flowerbed. Ben and Sam both voted for the manly primary colors. The red and yellow bulbs soon arrived by courier in an enormous cardboard box. There were lipstick-red Île-de-France tulips; fat, white Wildhof tulips; tiny, cream narcissus called Minnows and big ones called Yellow Mammoths. There were giant King Alfred daffodils; gorgeous white-and-orange narcissus called Tête à Tête; peppermint-striped Happy Generation tulips; and brilliant red anemones named His Excellency. According to the instructions, some bulbs bloomed in early spring and needed partial sun. Others emerged late, and preferred shade. How was I supposed to figure out what went where? The flowerbed got full sun in winter, weak sunlight in early spring and mostly shade in the summer. Meanwhile, some bulbs had to be planted three inches deep and four inches apart, others one-inch deep and half an inch apart. That was why I could never be a gardener. It required rulers and math. I stared glumly at my flourishing weeds. Then I threw away the directions and began digging wherever I pleased.

In a primal way, scrabbling in the earth under the warm autumn sun *was* healing. Around my two-hundredth bulb, it belatedly occurred to me that I was making myself an excellent target for a drive-by shooting. Just then a sleek Mercedes-Benz sedan pulled into my driveway. I brandished my trowel. At the same time, my journalist brain told me the car was way too fancy for a Quebec assassin who couldn't afford a spell-check.

It turned out to be my friend Joyce Johnston. A regal redhead, she was wearing a silk Burberry scarf draped around her neck. "What are you doing outside? Omigod! Am I in the line of fire?" she cried, removing her designer sunglasses.

Sheepishly, I told her that I *was* keeping an eye out for snipers, but I also had to get my bulbs in the ground. Joyce gave me a hug. Then she went around to the passenger side of her car and fetched a pot of *kalanchoe blossfeldiana*, a.k.a. Flaming Katy. It had tiny red-and-yellow flowers. It occurred to me that if I could keep it going until spring, it would be color-coordinated with my flowerbed. Not surprisingly, it stopped blooming after six months. Okay, I wasn't that great about watering it.

Two years later, Joyce's plant remains a reasonable shade of green. But the stems, once dense with fat, glossy leaves, have grown spindly. People who go through depression tend to be overwrought and I'm aware this is a florid metaphor, but I think of myself as the Flaming Katy; it has survived and so have I. Until very recently, I would not throw out the small greeting card that came with the plant. Stuck on a plastic spike embedded in the soil, it said, "With love, Joyce." It made me disproportionately happy that my friend had cared enough to stop by with a plant. The tiny card also reminded me that my employer had never sent anything.

As I write these words, my red and yellow tulips are blooming in profusion. Each spring, it is a marvelous healing moment, until Sam and his friends stomp the tulips to death while intercepting the basketballs that land on the flowerbed with percussive regularity. My doctor is a wise woman who prescribed a most inventive cure for paranoia. After I finished planting five hundred bulbs in the warm sunshine, I was no longer afraid of getting shot. I stopped skittering like a startled rabbit between my house and garage. As the days passed with no one blasting out my double-glazed, high-efficiency, thermal, white mullioned windows, the death threat began to recede.

I finally felt strong enough to phone the Manulife intervention specialist myself. She surprised me with a firm date for my return to work. "You should be off about six weeks," she said. "It shouldn't go beyond two months. You really need to resolve it."

I thought to myself that of course I would be back at the office very soon. There was no way it would take me two months to recover. After all, I felt so much better after digging in the earth. But then I felt a stab of anxiety. What if I wasn't better by then? I had worked with deadlines my whole career, but could I meet a wellness deadline? If I had had a broken hand, would the intervention specialist also impose a time limit on mending bones?

I asked how she was sure I would be okay within six weeks.

"You're not sick," she said. "I know because I've been doing disability assessment for thirty-two years."

CHAPTER 8

Death by a Thousand Cuts

Memory is the first casualty of depression. I forgot appointments. When I remembered them, I could no longer calculate when I had to leave the house in order to arrive at my destination on time. It was as if my brain had shut down. I found myself writing a mini-schedule for when to start getting dressed, when to walk out the door, how long the subway ride would take. Still, I often showed up too late or too early. Sometimes I forgot to show up at all and people thought I was rude, which made me feel worse.

I moved as if in a fog, uncertain of the time, the day or even the season. I once left the gas stove on when I went out. On one particularly bad day, I completely forgot to show up for eight parent-teacher meetings at school. One evening in a restaurant with friends, I suddenly realized I had forgotten my purse in the ladies' room. I jumped up from my chair and dashed back to the washroom. My purse was gone. Terribly upset, I returned to the table where my friends pointed to my purse, dangling from the back of my chair. From the looks on their faces, I knew they thought I was losing my mind. I am sure I was.

When I later read other accounts of depression, I was struck by the similarities. William Styron's own depression manifested all the classic symptoms: initial denial, confusion, memory lapses, self-loathing and failure of mental focus. He had no appetite. He was unable to sleep. He missed important appointments. In the midst of his clinical depression, he was honored with a literary award in Paris and flew over on the Concorde to attend the elegant presentation. He forgot, however, he was supposed to attend a lavish, post-ceremony luncheon with members of the Académie française. Right after accepting the twenty-five-thousand-dollar check, Styron clumsily explained to the donor that he had double-booked a lunch with his French publisher. Anyone who didn't know he was sick would assume he was a celebrity behaving badly. Indeed, the donor was enraged. Mortified, Styron clumsily attempted to apologize.

I blurted some words that a lifetime of general equilibrium, and a smug belief in the impregnability of my psychic health, had prevented me from believing I could ever utter; I was chilled as I heard myself speak them to this perfect stranger. "I'm sick," I said, "une problème psychiatrique."

For months, Styron had resisted the diagnosis. A few days before the prize ceremony, he finally acknowledged that he was severely depressed. "My dank joylessness was therefore all the more ironic because I had flown on a rushed four-day trip to Paris in order to accept an award which should have sparklingly restored my ego." A few hours after the ceremony, he lost the check and ended up on his knees, scrabbling underneath the table at a glittering brasserie. (Someone else in his party found it.) "Did I 'intend' to lose the money?" he wrote later. "Recently I had been deeply bothered that I was not deserving of the prize. I believe in the reality of the accidents we subconsciously perpetrate on ourselves, and so how easy it was for this loss to be not loss but a form of repudiation, offshoot of that self-loathing (depression's premier badge) by which I was persuaded that I could not be worthy of the prize..."

I wasn't merely forgetting appointments and losing my purse (or thinking I had). I also have no memory of what was happening with my family. What did we do for Thanksgiving that first year? Halloween? Did Ben and Sam go out at all? Dressed up as what?

That November I forgot Norman's sixty-third birthday.

"Sorry," I had said, ten days late.

"That's okay."

"Really? You're okay with that?"

"I'd just as soon forget it myself."

Norman, a generous and forgiving human, genuinely didn't mind—even though he knew he would have heard about it endlessly if he'd forgotten *my* birthday. My husband is a man of few words. After thirty years of marriage, his quiet acceptance of my mercurial moods spoke volumes about his constancy and love.

We met at a Merry Marxmas party at the home of a left-wing Canadian teacher in Beijing. Norman was dressed in a blue Mao suit, a cap pulled low over his forehead. I'm embarrassed to admit this—I partly blame the Mao cap and his impeccable Mandarin—but at first I thought he was Chinese. After I belatedly realized he was a nice Jewish boy from New York—and emphatically not Chinese—we continued to converse in Mandarin, even later when we began dating, perhaps because we were both staunch supporters of the revolution. Luckily for our marriage, we both became disillusioned with Maoism at about the same time (at which point we gradually switched to speaking English). The funny thing is, while we abandoned the ideology, we retained the righteous stubbornness.

Like me, Norman was idealistic and principled. He believed in integrity and human rights and speaking truth to power. He was fiercely supportive when I was ill. He never once told me to suck it up and get back to the office. He never once doubted I was sick. With him by my side, I knew I had an ally when I could no longer stand my ground alone.

Despite Norman's support, I kept losing weight. I cried all the time. Even with sleeping pills and the occasional tranquilizer, I was not sleeping well. My libido vanished. I got lost driving through familiar neighborhoods. Then I read the fine print on Ativan and realized I shouldn't be at the wheel at all. I stopped driving.

Depression is insidious. It permeates the atmosphere of the home, affecting the whole family. Occasionally it occurred to me that I was no longer functioning as a wife or mother, but I was incapable of doing anything about it. I had already stopped writing. Now I lost my role within the family, which deepened my sense of loss. The death threat had destabilized us all.

"Do you think the police will be able to protect us?" Ben asked.

"Yes, of course," I said, but my voice quavered.

Whenever Sam was home alone at night, he avoided the main floor. We didn't know it at the time, but my younger son had stashed a baseball bat under his bedroom bookcase. One day, he broached the topic of hand-to-hand combat. "What if he's already in the house? Should I hide? Or should I phone 911?"

I advised Sam to run out of the house. Then I added, "But if you're trapped, call 911. Make sure you say we're on the priority list."

"What if he hears me calling 911?"

"Then shout: 'the police are on the way!'"

My thirteen-year-old and I were talking about "him" as if he were real. We plotted our strategy as if a home invasion was imminent, as if a flesh-and-blood assassin was on his way to attack us. I knew I was transmitting my paranoia and anxiety to my children, but I couldn't help myself. Only Norman remained calm.

It's fashionable these days to dump on Freud. But after I recovered, it was a revelation to read "Mourning and Melancholia." Freud writes that both grief and depression are triggered by loss and have identical reactions: lack of interest in sex and food, memory problems and an inability to feel joy.

However, melancholia, from the Greek word for "sadness," is different from mourning in one key way. Melancholia also results, Freud says, in the sudden "lowering of the self-regarding feelings to a degree that finds utterance in self-reproaches and self-revilings." In other words, when you're depressed, your self-esteem plunges. Certainly it happened to me, even though my self-esteem and confidence had always been robust.

Patricia Kirby, the retired Toronto psychotherapist, calls this severe loss of self-esteem, "death by a thousand cuts, real or imagined." In ancient China, death by a thousand cuts was an actual form of capital punishment. Called *lingchi*, it was meted out for the most heinous crimes: treason, patricide, matricide, or mass murder of a single clan. The last known execution by a thousand cuts took place in 1904 in a public square in Beijing. It was formally abolished in 1905, in the waning years of the last imperial dynasty. In death by *lingchi*, the executioner would methodically slice off portions of the body, beginning with the eyes, ears, nose, tongue, fingers and toes. After a few main cuts, the executioner would stab the victim in the heart before continuing to slice up and dismember the corpse. The intent was not to inflict pain per se, but to cut up the body into many pieces. This was the most terrible punishment of all because the Chinese believed in Confucianism, the reigning ideology, which held that one's body had to be kept intact for the afterlife.

Sure, I wasn't in China, and it wasn't 1904. I wasn't even bleeding. But it still felt like a death by a thousand cuts. The worst cut of all was being silenced. Freedom of speech was intrinsic to my profession, my job, my identity, everything I cared about. I began to turn inward. My world narrowed to a pinhole. Scrutinizing myself in my bathroom mirror, it seemed I had aged. There were new wrinkles, deep shadows under my eyes. An unexplained rash covered my arms and legs, burning whenever I showered. I was convinced my hair was turning white and falling out. I developed a twitch under my left eye. I hoped no one noticed. I didn't want to look like a crazy person.

Why the left eye? Why not the right?

I was now seeing Dr. Au every week. She would listen for an hour as I recited a litany of woe—rashes and twitches and sleepless nights. "I'm afraid you're falling into a depression," she said.

I rejected the diagnosis. I was sad, but I was *not* clinically depressed. I didn't pause to consider why I doubted my doctor. If she had told me I had the flu or a cracked rib, I would not have disputed her conclusion. If she had said I had cancer, I might have waited for the test results. (But then, so would Dr. Au.) That's the unsettling nature of mental illness. Until advances in brain science bring full objectivity to the diagnosis of conditions such as depression, patients themselves will invariably question whether they are actually ill.

At my next visit, my doctor said, "I'd like to put you on antidepressants."

I burst into tears. So far I had accepted the occasional tranquilizer, but I remained fearful of antidepressants. What if they permanently changed my personality? What about the side effects? What if they made me drool? Were they addictive? What if I went on them, and couldn't get off without going crazy? I could already hear the jeers. *Oh, she's off her meds.* At the same time, I wondered why I objected so strenuously. No one would feel embarrassed about taking pills for heart disease or diabetes.

This is how I analyzed my condition: I wasn't *depressed*. I just needed a bit more time off. I could work through this without going on medication. But I didn't even want to discuss medication with my doctor. Instead, I choked back sobs and mopped my eyes and my doctor dropped the subject. On the subway I cried all the way home. Words like "madness," "lunacy" and "insanity" ricocheted in my head. My fellow passengers averted their eyes.

Until a century ago, depression was known as "melancholia." The word came from the Greek: *melas* for "black" and *khole* for "bile." The ancients believed that personality was formed from the body's four basic "humors": blood, phlegm, yellow bile and black bile. Those with an excess of blood, the sanguine types, had a ruddy complexion and an optimistic disposition. Phlegmatic ones were calm and unemotional. Choleric types had an excess of choler—yellow bile—and were bad-tempered and irritable. Melancholics, who had too much black bile, were gloomy. (An early theory was that excessive black bile also caused cancer.)

For centuries, everyone used the term "melancholy." Then in 1904, Adolf Meyer, the Swiss-born president of the American Psychiatric Association, suggested switching to a less emotive word: depression. Styron writes:

Melancholia ... was usurped by a noun with a bland tonality and lacking any magisterial presence, used indifferently to describe an economic decline or a rut in the ground, a true wimp of a word for such a major illness. Nonetheless, for over seventy-five years the word has slithered innocuously through the language like a slug, leaving little trace of its intrinsic malevolence and preventing, by its very insipidity, a general awareness of the horrible intensity of the disease when out of control.

Depression is not a benign illness. It is a form of madness. I lost my rationality, sense of reality, proportionality. Everything happened, quite literally, in my head. Under stress, my brain's biochemistry changed. There was too much cortisol, too little serotonin and not enough noradrenalin. ("Adrenalin" and "noradrenalin" are the British names for what in the United States are known as "epinephrine" and "norepinephrine" respectively.) The imbalance was putting my body into overdrive, shutting down non-emergency systems and affecting my lungs, liver, kidneys, heart, gastro-intestinal function and immune system. My family doctor noted that my blood pressure was elevated for the first time in my life.

Although depression is indisputably biochemical, no biopsy, MRI scan or biochemical test can confirm a doctor's diagnosis. Instead, psychiatrists and family physicians rely on a list of nine symptoms, devised back in the 1860s by the superintendents of the first insane asylums in America. Their notes form the basis of the bible of modern psychiatry, the *Diagnostic and Statistical Manual of Mental Disorders*. The fourth edition, known as *DSM-IV*, lists the following symptoms:

- depressed mood
- diminished interest or pleasure in normal daily activities
- loss of appetite and significant weight loss without dieting, or overeating and rapid weight gain
- inability to sleep or excessive sleeping
- psychomotor retardation or agitation
- fatigue, loss of energy
- feelings of worthlessness and inappropriate guilt
- diminished ability to think or concentrate, indecisiveness
- recurrent thoughts of death or suicidal ideation, suicide attempt or specific plan

To meet the diagnosis of clinical depression, you must have five or more symptoms on the list and they must persist for at least two weeks or more. A day or two of feeling down doesn't count.

I had eight of nine symptoms. And by the time Dr. Au was pressing me to take antidepressants, my symptoms had already lasted two months. Only the last symptom, suicide ideation, was absent. As time went on, however, I would occasionally think of killing myself. I felt embarrassed about that and told no one at the time, not even the psychiatrist who would later take over my treatment. In fact, I remember assuring him, quite cheerily at my first appointment, that I wasn't going to kill myself.

The intervention specialist from Manulife phoned again. It was now close to the six-week limit she had specified as the maximum length of my sick leave. Unfortunately I still felt incapable of doing my job. I dreaded the idea of going out to interview anyone. I didn't think I could write a coherent story. The thought of a deadline made me nauseous.

"How will I know I am ready to go back?" I asked nervously.

"You'll be just fine," she said reassuringly and suggested I see a therapist to prepare for my return to work. "They can help you with coping strategies."

Like Joseph K. in *The Trial*, who would never come face to face with his judge, I would never meet my intervention specialist. For the next two years, she would remain a faceless, disembodied voice, communicating only by snail mail and telephone, not even by email. She would never provide an address of any kind except for a corporate post-office box. I had no idea what city she lived in. If I wanted to contact her, I had only a toll-free number. It was, well, Kafkaesque. The intervention specialist controlled my fate, my health, my job, my sick pay, my very identity. But what was I to her? Was I just another file, a bit of paperwork outsourced by my employer to be processed through the vast computer system of another major corporation? Or did she look forward to the day when I was healthy, so her job would be done and the file closed?

After talking to the specialist on the phone that day, I dutifully booked a therapy appointment through the *Globe*'s employee-assistance program. To my surprise, although I lived in a city of four million people (presumably with many, many therapists), I was given a slot to talk by phone to someone on the West Coast, three time zones away. At the appointed hour, I dialed yet another toll-free number and was immediately connected.

The therapist began by asking about my mood. Did I feel downhearted and sad? Did I have trouble sleeping? Did I awaken in the morning feeling fresh and vigorous? He asked me to tell him what had triggered my depression. I disliked recounting my long and complicated tale of woe yet again and I didn't like talking over the phone to a stranger, but I tried my best.

"It sounds like a real complex situation," he said, when I finished. "It's natural to go through anxiety and some depression. There are a lot of people walking around with post-traumatic stress. Your space has been violated."

I told him I didn't feel ready to go back to work and asked how I should prepare myself for my first day back. The jargon spilled forth. The "strategy," he said, was to find "meaning out of all this." I had suffered "emotional abuse." I needed to "re-establish" my self-esteem. "We have to disengage sometime," he added. "It's a no-win situation, but we have to survive. You're off the scoreboard with stress. But we are not supposed to recommend time away from work."

My hour was up. If I understood him correctly, I was suffering from anxiety, depression and post-traumatic stress—but I still had to go back to work. Somewhere in my barely functioning brain, the reporter in me found it fascinating how frankly he admitted: "we are not supposed to recommend time away from work."

"The test of a first-rate intelligence is the ability to hold two opposed ideas in the mind at the same time, and still retain the ability to function," F. Scott Fitzgerald wrote in *The Crack-Up*. "One should, for example, be able to see that things are hopeless and yet be determined to make them otherwise."

Were things hopeless at my workplace? I was determined to return, but as the days passed in a blur with no improvement in my mood, I lost track of time. I realized it was late fall only when I noticed brown and red leaves on the sidewalk. Then Gigi phoned with another getaway idea.

"You could take Dad somewhere warm," she said.

So I booked my father and myself a suite at a golf resort in Scottsdale, Arizona, even though neither of us golfed. All that mattered was that the sun shone nine days out of ten. I looked forward to spending an entire week with my father. At the same time, I wondered what we would do all day, an unhappy daughter and a half-blind, half-deaf octogenarian father.

We had never been a demonstrative family. I don't remember Dad ever hugging or kissing us as children. He never propped up our self-esteem. Yet I knew his love for us was unconditional. I knew, too, he was thrilled when I, alone among his children, learned to read, write and speak Chinese. He was proud when I was hired as the news assistant for *The New York Times* bureau in Beijing. He knew my ambition had been to return to China as a foreign correspondent, so in 1988 when *The Globe and Mail* appointed me Beijing bureau chief, he said approvingly, "You got what you always wanted." It was the highest praise.

Mom taught us to cook, clean house, cut hair, mend a sock, pack a suitcase and whistle a happy tune. Dad taught us how to manage money. When I received my first paycheck from the Montreal *Gazette*, he recommended investments and gave me a lump sum to get me started. I saved and invested and saved more, ending up financially secure.

When Dad and I emerged from the airport into the brilliant Arizona sunshine, we both exhaled with pleasure. My father, who loved anything free, was thrilled to find a lemonade dispenser in the hotel lobby. He was even happier when the concierge upgraded us to a deluxe, handicapped-accessible, one-bedroom suite with a dining-room table that seated eight. The only imperfection was the bathroom, which had two doors and no locks. I tried to institute a system.

"Dad, how about we keep both doors open when we're not using the bathroom, and close both doors when we are?"

My father nodded but, at eighty-six, he wasn't into systems. He always left both doors ajar.

We also argued companionably about who would get the bedroom.

"You take it." I told him.

"No, you take it." He pointed out that being half-deaf and half-blind were ideal conditions for falling asleep in the living room. Filial piety, however, would not allow me to let my father sleep on the sofa bed. So around eight o'clock each night, he would retreat into the bedroom. Alone in the living room, I would watch television, hour after hour, something I never did at home. When I finally switched off the lights, I couldn't fall asleep.

My mind would race through a labyrinth of guilt. I kept going over and over the Dawson story and the backlash. Like a plot device in an Ian McEwan novel, one random occurrence had set off an inexorable chain of events and everything changed. All paths seemed to lead to the same unanswerable question: what had I done wrong? I was in the grip of a ruminative cycle, what the blogger Jonah Lehrer calls "a recursive loop of woe." "Ruminate," from the Latin for "chew again," describes the way cattle chew, swallow, regurgitate and re-chew their food. In psychiatric terms, rumination means obsessing about a problem, thereby reinforcing and prolonging the negative mood. Ruminating is the thought process that defines depression.

In my haste to give Dad the bedroom, I had forgotten he was an early riser. Each morning, he awakened at dawn, just as I was falling asleep. He would emerge from the bedroom, snap on a couple of lights in the kitchen and attempt to make a cup of coffee. Water roared from the tap. Spoons rattled. Stoneware cups crashed against granite counters. Fifteen feet away, I covered my face with a pillow and realized how much my teenage boys suffered whenever I shook them awake at the crack of noon.

I have never been a do-nothing vacationer. After trying out all three pools at the hotel, I told Dad I wanted to hike Camelback Mountain. He was worried I would get lost or killed and insisted on coming along. That was touching considering it was unclear how he could have rescued me from a bushy-bearded, axe-wielding mountain man. Even with his cane,

Dad could walk no more than half a block on flat terrain. At any rate, the mountain trail, in the middle of Phoenix, turned out to be far from deserted. Lycra-clad hikers brandished high-tech canes, one in each hand, like cross-country skiers. They pushed past me like New Yorkers on the subway at rush hour, barking, "Excuse me! Excuse me!"

After a two-hour hike, I found my father waiting patiently at the bottom of the mountain. He was sitting on a rock, head sunk, dehydrated and tired. After that, he stayed in the suite to watch football while I explored the desert alone. Each day, I rushed back to have lunch with him and then left him alone, puffing a cigar on our private patio. Melodramatically, I worried that every moment together might be our last. The week slipped by. I wanted to tell him how much I loved him, but the years of not expressing our feelings had left me tongue-tied. Dad's silence was oddly therapeutic. Once when I alluded to my problems, he said gruffly, "Don't *worry*." The week in Arizona taught me a fundamental lesson in parenting. Caring doesn't have to mean talking, talking, talking. It can also mean standing beside your kids, even your adult kids, in their moment of need. Sometimes just being there is everything.

I was a teenager when my mother mentioned she had once felt like killing herself. I was upset, of course. But I changed the subject because I didn't want to know anything about it. After I had been through depression myself, I mentioned Mom's long-ago crisis with the family. Gigi said Mom had told her about being depressed, but nothing about contemplating suicide. Like me, my sister had shied away from asking for details. As for Dad, he had known nothing at all. He thought about it for a moment. "It's a lot of work looking after four kids."

Arizona's sunshine and endless desert were healing. One day I took Dad for a pedicure in Sun City. He discovered that he loved soaking his feet in warm, scented water and having a pretty young woman buff his toenails. Emboldened, I suggested a mid-morning excursion to Scottsdale Fashion Square. I didn't tell him it was the largest shopping mall in the southwestern United States. "Okay," said Dad, who hates shopping.

For some reason, buying things, especially shoes, suddenly made me happy. Normally, Dad would frown and mutter about how ridiculous it was that anyone needed more than two pairs at any given time. This time when I said I wanted to duck into Macy's, he said again, "Okay." Then he flopped down on a sofa strategically placed just outside the store's main doors.

When I emerged an hour later with three new pairs of shoes, he didn't scowl. He listened while I enthused about them: sage-green suede loafers, black microfiber heels, high-heeled Ralph Lauren mules. He even tried to look interested. I was supposed to be taking care of Dad, but he was taking care of me. It was his way of telling me he loved me: waiting for his sad, forgetful daughter while she shopped for shoes she didn't need.

CHAPTER 9

Despair Beyond Despair

I felt somewhat better after my Arizona trip and hoped I could soon return to the newsroom. But the psychological relief evaporated the day after I got back. First the union told me that human resources had wrapped up its investigation—without ever having interviewed me. Then a courier delivered a letter with the results of that investigation. HR was blaming me and putting a disciplinary note in my personnel file. The note said:

> *Every reasonable effort was made to protect you as a journalist and to protect the reputation of The Globe and Mail during this difficult time.... You went far beyond your request to speak only about the personal attacks on you and your family and used your position as a Globe and Mail reporter to question the Prime Minister and the Premier of Quebec.*

I divided into two again: the person falling apart and the ironic observer who wondered: *what kind of newspaper scolds its reporter for criticizing politicians?*

William Styron, who has called depression the "despair beyond despair," discussed the ability of a depressive to split into two. "A phenomenon that a number of people have noted while in deep depression is the sense of being accompanied by a second self—a wraithlike observer who, not sharing the dementia of his double, is able to watch with dispassionate curiosity as his companion struggles against the oncoming disaster..."

After writing *War and Peace*, Tolstoy himself endured a depression so severe, a plunge in his self-esteem so precipitous, that he felt unworthy of his inherited wealth and gave most of it away. That experience with depression influenced his later novel, *Anna Karenina*, in which he described this same phenomenon of splitting into two. In the scene where Anna confesses her infidelity to her husband, he wrote, Anna "was not simply miserable, she began to feel alarm at the new emotional condition, never experienced before, in which she found herself. She felt as though everything was beginning to be doubled in her soul, just as objects sometimes appear doubled to overtired eyes."

The two-page, single-spaced disciplinary note—the first in my career—shattered me. In my hyper-anxious state, I considered it ominous, the first step toward dismissal. I knew that employers who wanted to get rid of someone first created a paper trail. Worse, I felt that I had been found guilty, or condemned, or whatever you want to call it, without ever having had the chance to defend myself. Naively, I had waited weeks for the HR vice-president to interview me, to hear my side of events. She never bothered to call. Had there even been an investigation at all?

Most painful of all was the realization that the disciplinary note formalized the gag order—and made it permanent:

It is critically important that we work together as the reputation of both you and the newspaper are important matters which need consultation.... Further, you are not to speak with or otherwise provide information to any other media organization regarding the operation ... of The Globe and Mail without obtaining prior written approval..."

The note concluded: "A copy of this letter will be placed in your personnel file."

I would never be able to speak about what had happened to me. My anxiety grew. I cried many times a day. Normally, tears bring catharsis. Now they consumed and exhausted me. Gloom enveloped me, transforming everything to shadows, muting sights, sounds and smells.

A day later, the Manulife intervention specialist phoned. She seemed annoyed that I had gone to Arizona without her permission. I explained that my doctor had recommended travel. I added, lamely, that I didn't realize I was supposed to seek approval. The specialist was more concerned, however, with setting a date for my return. She suggested I start with half days. I explained that working at half-speed wasn't feasible in a newsroom with daily deadlines. By the time I finished a story, it might no longer be news. More significantly, I explained I still couldn't write. I told her I had been testing myself by trying in vain to get back into a book manuscript I had started earlier.

As I have said, I had rarely been sick and I had no experience of dealing with human resources, let alone an intervention specialist. Looking back, I think this was the moment when I might have inadvertently planted a poisonous seed, a seed that would soon flower into full-blown suspicion and mistrust. What did the Manulife specialist hear—that I *was* writing my book? And what did she report back, if anything, to my newspaper? How did management interpret the information?

The company knew I had two books on the go because six months earlier I had applied for, and been routinely granted, two short unpaid book leaves. I had completed the first leave just before the Dawson shootings. My second leave was scheduled to start after the Christmas holidays. Depending on what the intervention specialist reported, management could easily have pieced the evidence together this way: *she's a disgruntled diva, in a snit after the editor-in-chief's column criticized her. Now she's calling in sick so she can write her books while drawing down sick pay.*

Who knows what my employer thought? What's clear is that many companies fail to recognize mental illness. Or if they recognize it, they hate the uncertainty and potential hit to the bottom line. After I told the Manulife intervention specialist I still couldn't write, that I'd been testing myself by trying to write my book and couldn't, she repeated, "You're not sick. Your leave would not be supported."

Again she told me that six weeks was the maximum I could be off sick. I'd already been off five weeks. It meant I'd have to be back in the office, working as a reporter, in a week. I hung up the phone, burst into tears and stuck a tranquilizer under my tongue. How could I go back when I still couldn't write? How could I *prove* I couldn't write? What if I went back to the newsroom in this state and was fired for zero productivity? So many surreal things had happened I hardly knew what to expect next.

Trembling, I opened my filing cabinet and fished out my benefits brochure. To my surprise, I discovered that short-term disability maxed out at six *months*, not six weeks. Why had the intervention specialist told me, with such certainty, that my sick leave could only last six weeks? And what did she mean—my leave "would not be supported"? I phoned my cousin-in-law, Colleen, who is a lawyer and former president of a multi-billion-dollar pension fund.

"It means they will cut off your salary and benefits."

Norman was outraged. He did not believe the newspaper could legally cut off my sick pay. I realized I faced a stark choice. I could stand up for my right to be ill or I could go back to work. "Maybe I should just go back to work," I told him tearfully.

"You can't go back while you're still sick," Norman said. "Not if your doctor says you can't."

Depression is "the flaw in love," wrote Andrew Solomon. I was in love with journalism and it would break my heart. I had worked at the *Globe* for nearly twenty years. In that time I had been reliable and trustworthy. I had been given the toughest assignments. I had delivered the kind of stories that drew readers and sold papers. So how did I go, practically overnight, from a valued corporate asset to—how to put this delicately—a bag of shit?

Was this, as I felt it was during my depression, happening only to me? Or might there be something bigger going on? I had always been loyal to my company. But are companies still loyal to employees? Do they dump you the moment you become a problem?

In the 1950s and 1960s, the workforce was stable. That was the era of the "organization man," when men (yes, *men*) joined a company and stayed for life. Then out of the blue, the world changed. Competition went global. Corporations no longer wanted managers who maintained the status quo. Instead they sought out those "who could shake the trees, rattle cages and get things done quickly," according to Paul Babiak and Richard D. Hare in their book, *Snakes in Suits: When Psychopaths Go to Work*. Babiak is an industrial psychologist and president of HRBackOffice, an executive coaching and consulting firm in New York. Hare is a retired professor of psychology at the University of British Columbia and the creator of the standard diagnostic tool for psychopathy used by the FBI and other law enforcement organizations.

Babiak and Hare pointed out that rattling cages—a massive layoff, for instance—often enhances the bottom line. Management and shareholders applaud such brutality and call it efficiency. Indeed, bad news for employees is often good news for the company's stock price. The same measures that make companies mean often make them lean. But when bullying on the job is framed as tough management, workplaces become toxic. And absenteeism, low morale and high turnover often cancel out any bottom-line savings. Currently one in every twelve employees in Canada takes medication for depression and other mental-health conditions. Each day, half a million Canadian workers are off sick with mental-health problems.

I was about to become a statistic. At my next appointment, I told Dr. Au that Manulife said I wasn't sick and had ordered me to report to work. If I didn't comply, my sick pay would be halted. I began to sob. She looked concerned. "You're not better yet. I'm afraid you will get worse if you go back prematurely," she said. "You need to consider taking antidepressants."

Tears coursed down my cheeks. Was I sick or not? Who was right, the insurer or my doctor? I could walk and talk. I wasn't lying in bed. But I couldn't write. If only I could have a brief respite from the ultimatums and threats, I thought, perhaps I could recover. Yet if I stayed out, my sick pay would stop. I said none of this aloud. My doctor sat silently, watching me.

"I'm afraid you're getting depressed," she said, repeating what she had told me at previous appointments.

Acceptance of diagnosis is one of the most difficult aspects of the illness. It is also the first step to recovery. At my last appointment, I wouldn't even discuss going on medication. Now my doctor handed me a free starter package of Effexor. She knew that I couldn't resist free samples of anything, even antidepressants. I accepted it, tucked it in my bag and said I would think about it. Then Dr. Au wrote another sick note, extending my leave until early January. At home, I faxed it to the human-resources department. A few days later, on December 5, I received another couriered letter from my employer.

"We require you to return to work Wednesday, December 6 at 9 A.M."

CHAPTER 10

Melancholia Through the Ages

Depression has probably been with us since the first, sad cavewoman crawled into her cave and refused to come out.

Originally the illness implied no dishonor. Around 1500 B.C., clinical depression was matter-of-factly mentioned in the Ebers Papyrus, one of the oldest medical documents in the world. In the eighth century, Muslim physicians established the first psychiatric hospitals and insane asylums in Baghdad, Cairo and Fes, Morocco. In ancient Greece, Socrates believed melancholia was a consequence of overly rigorous philosophizing. Hippocrates thought it was a malady of the brain. Aristotle, who very likely suffered from it himself, linked it to brilliant achievement. "All men who have attained excellence in philosophy, in poetry, in art and in politics, even Socrates and Plato, had a melancholic habitus. Indeed some suffered even from melancholic disease," he wrote in the fourth century B.C.

Over the centuries, however, depression acquired a stigma. In medieval Europe, Christian doctrine held that the soul was a divine gift so that anyone full of God's grace had to be, by holy definition, happy. Therefore anyone unhappy had to be lacking God's grace. They were, quite literally, *dis*graceful. By that same holy definition, depressives were sinners. You felt bad, ergo you *were* bad.

By the sixth century, suicide, the final act of a depressive, became a mortal sin and a secular crime. The ultimate sinner, of course, was Judas Iscariot, the apostle who betrayed Jesus and afterward hanged himself. In 1562, the Church began denying suicides a Christian burial in consecrated ground. By 1693, even attempting suicide became a religious crime, punishable by excommunication.

Secular laws reinforced this prejudice. Anyone who took their own life forfeited all worldly possessions, not only their own, but their entire family's, to the state. Suddenly, there was an urgent economic motive for family members to cover up any trace of the "crime." This, I believe, is the beginning of the furtiveness and guilt that now surrounds the illness, the historic roots of the stigma. Today, even though we don't know exactly why we feel ashamed, many of us go to great lengths to keep our depression a secret. That is why I felt so self-conscious with Dr. Au's receptionist and the reason so many people today feel ashamed about seeing a psychiatrist or letting anyone know they are taking antidepressants.

By the time of the Inquisition, melancholia became known as *acedia*, a word from ancient Greek meaning "without care." *Acedia* manifested itself as listlessness, sluggishness, torpor and exhaustion—in other words, the inability to get out of bed. By the thirteenth century, *acedia* became known as sloth and was listed as one of the seven deadly sins. The prejudice had come full circle: anyone too lazy to get out of bed was, again by holy definition, a sinner.

During the Renaissance, the stigma temporarily disappeared as philosophers venerated sadness and romanticized the illness. Like Aristotle, they believed melancholia was the price genius paid for inspiration and insight; it was a prerequisite for the artistic life. During the Elizabethan era, this romantic link made the illness almost fashionable. By the 1600s, Richard Napier, a physician in Great Linford, Buckinghamshire, found that even though his practice was devoted to farming families, a disproportionate 40 percent of his melancholic patients were aristocrats. Were the philosophers of the Renaissance right to link depression and creativity? Numerous modern studies have shown that creative types suffer significantly higher rates of mood disorders than the general population, a phenomenon noted in *Touched with Fire: Manic-Depressive Illness and the Artistic Temperament*, by Kay Redfield Jamison, a professor of psychiatry who has written extensively about her own struggle with manic-depression.

Unfortunately, the stigma resurfaced in the eighteenth century. The Age of Reason was the worst time in history to be perceived as lacking the capacity to reason. In France, female depressives were incarcerated alongside prostitutes and epileptics. They were treated as wild animals and chained to prison walls. Reformist physicians began crusading for a more humane, psychological approach. In 1795, Dr. Philippe Pinel famously unchained the depressives at Pitié-Salpêtrière, a former gunpowder factory that is now the largest hospital in Paris. (The hospital is famous also as the place Sigmund Freud studied psychiatric patients in 1895 and where Princess Diana was pronounced dead in 1997.)

In America "sloth" remained a sin. Puritans in the New World brought with them the work ethic of the Old World. They believed that anyone who could not get out of bed had to be possessed. "Some Devil is often very Busy with the poor Melancholicks," wrote Cotton Mather, an influential figure at the Salem witch trials. "Yea, there is often a Degree of Diabolical

Possession in the Melancholy." By the nineteenth century, attitudes in America began changing. The popular exhortation of the day, "Go West, young man!" symbolized the pioneering spirit. But doctors, fretting that the unbridled freedom of the American Way would promote mental instability, considered it their patriotic duty to treat melancholics. Public opinion—and tax revenues—supported the doctors. In an era before government-funded public education, almost every state levied taxes to support at least one insane asylum.

This was the tolerant environment in which Abraham Lincoln ran for the presidency. He frequently talked of suicide while he was on the stump. He wept in public and often sat with his chin sunk against his chest. "His melancholy dripped from him as he walked," said his law partner, William Herndon. Remarkably, Lincoln's chronic depression was never a reason to question his fitness for office. On the contrary, public knowledge of it enhanced his political career. "His moods consistently provoked empathy, assistance, and admiration," writes Joshua Wolf Shenk in *Lincoln's Melancholy, How Depression Challenged a President and Fueled His Greatness*.

In 1860, a Democratic newspaper broke the story of the Republican candidate's first mental breakdown, but not as scandalmongering or an attempt to demolish Lincoln's chances. Instead the story was presented favorably, as a tale of triumph over adversity. At a critical juncture in American history, Lincoln's ability to deal with melancholia became an issue of character, a *positive* trait.

A century later, public attitudes had regressed. In 1972 Edmund Muskie's apparent tears at a press conference derailed his bid for the Democratic presidential nomination. Then Thomas Eagleton, a vice-presidential candidate, revealed that he had been hospitalized for depression and treated with electroshock therapy. The ensuing outcry forced Eagleton to quit the race. In the fallout, Richard Nixon, the Republican incumbent, was re-elected president in a landslide. Ironically, Nixon had suffered from a depression, too, but had kept it a secret. Following the hostile public reaction to his 1970 bombing of Cambodia, he had been medicating himself with Dilantin, a mood-altering prescription drug. His depression was revealed only in 2000, with the publication Anthony Summers's *The Arrogance of Power: The Secret World of Richard Nixon*.

These days, politicians are permitted, like Lincoln, to shed a few tears in public. In 2008, commentators approved when Hillary Clinton's eyes welled up. The polls soared when Barack Obama wiped away tears on news of his grandmother death, hours before he went on to win the presidency. Today, crying is seen to humanize a political candidate. Emotion is one thing, emotional instability another. Any whiff of mental illness still would almost certainly destroy a presidential campaign.

Similarly, many professional careers would be ruined, or at least, people perceive that they would be. In a survey of psychiatrists by the Michigan Psychiatric Society, half said they would medicate themselves secretly rather than have mental illness recorded on their charts. This is despite the fact that doctors are twice as likely to commit suicide as others. And until recently, the U.S. Federal Aviation Administration forced any pilot taking antidepressants to retire. In 2010 the FAA softened its stance slightly, allowing pilots to take one of four approved antidepressants if they can demonstrate they have been satisfactorily treated with the drug for at least twelve months. The FAA said it would accept Prozac, Zoloft, Celexa and Lexapro or their generic equivalents.

While the Canadian Forces recognize both mental and physical sacrifice, the U.S. military does not. In 2009 the Pentagon stated it would continue to award a Purple Heart to soldiers who bleed as a result of enemy action, but would not extend eligibility to victims of post-traumatic stress disorder. And yet the emotional toll exacted by invisible wounds can be lethal. In 2009 the number of suicides reported by the U.S. Army rose to the highest level in thirty years. In the first six months of 2009 alone, there were 129 confirmed or suspected suicides, "more than the number of American soldiers who died in combat during the same period," The New York Times reported. And these figures did not include soldiers who had left the service.

The mystery, however, is why the stigma rebounded with a vengeance after Lincoln's time. I blame the advent of laissez-faire capitalism, the nineteenth-century ideology that held that the state should not interfere in transactions between individuals. In Cotton Mather's time, one's fate depended in part on the devil, an unpredictable, uncontrollable outside force. Under laissez-faire capitalism, the individual suddenly became wholly responsible for his or her own fate. For instance, under this creed, The Economist solemnly argued it would be a violation of natural law for the government to provide free food during the Irish famine of 1846 to 1849, a catastrophe in which more than 1.5 million starved to death.

By the 1950s, the ideology of unbridled capitalism had elevated the individual to the pinnacle of society. At the same time, capitalism undermined the growth of social-welfare systems that might have mitigated its more pernicious effects. In her 1957 novel Atlas Shrugged, the twentieth-century Russian-American philosopher Ayn Rand contended that the highest moral purpose of life is the pursuit of individual happiness. The subtext: if you aren't happy, it's your own fault.

Today individuals are expected to take control of everything from their personal net worth to their body weight. Self-help books have flooded the market. Glossy magazines run headlines such as "GET A GOLD MEDAL BODY!"; "EIGHT SECRETS TO BEING THE LIFE OF THE PARTY!"; and "GET THE JOB YOU WANT—NOW!" The message to all the losers waiting in the supermarket-checkout line: if only you had a proper work ethic, you, too, could attain *Success! Wealth! Beauty! Happiness!* Above all, *Happiness!*

It's an attitude that leads us right back to the full-of-grace Middle Ages. In the twenty-first century, as in medieval times, we continue to conflate melancholy and sloth. If you can't get out of bed, you're a loser, you have a bad work ethic, you lack ambition, you're pathetic, *you're gonna be poor for the rest of your life*. All these centuries later, our attitude toward people who are feeling down remains harsh. They violate our bedrock Western belief that you can always pull up your socks and get back to work at improving your lot in life. A depressive, in essence, personifies the rejection of the American dream.

Despite their vastly different culture and religion, the ancient Chinese approached depression with much the same tolerance as the ancient Greeks. But instead of an excess of black bile, the Chinese blamed an irregularity of vital energy known as *qi* (pronounced *chee*). Two millennia ago, the medical classic *Inner Canon of the Yellow Emperor* stated, "In a patient full of grief and sadness, the *qi* becomes depressed and does not move." In the seventh century, a treatise known as *A Discussion of the Symptoms and Origins of Disease* (Zhubing Yuanhou Lun) attributed melancholia to "knotted *qi*." By the fourteenth century, Chinese doctors had linked mind and body, though perhaps a bit too much. "Once there is depression, all kinds of diseases will develop. Therefore, all of the body's diseases are caused by depression," wrote the physician, Zhu Danxi.

Unlike in the West, there was no religious proscription against suicide in Asia. In fact, samurai in medieval Japan were revered for choosing death over dishonor. During World War II, kamikaze pilots were the original suicide bombers. Back home they were venerated for their sacrifice in deliberately crashing planes into Allied warships. The legacy lingers today. In 2007, when a Japanese cabinet minister facing a bribery probe hanged himself, the governor of Tokyo praised the dead man as a "true samurai."

In imperial China, suicide was also morally permissible and even praised. In 278 B.C., the poet-official Qu Yuan remonstrated a corrupt emperor by clasping a rock to his chest and drowning himself in a river, an act that was considered a righteous response to a difficult situation. While the evil emperor is long forgotten, Qu Yuan's sacrifice is still commemorated today through annual dragon-boat races in China and around the world. In dynastic China, whenever an emperor was overthrown, Confucian officials would emulate Qu Yuan, committing suicide in droves. "The idea was the loyal official would not serve the new regime," said Timothy Brook, professor of history at the University of British Columbia.

After Mao Zedong led the Communist Party to victory in 1949, he denounced China's ancient culture. Instead, at least in the early years of the People's Republic, he looked to the Soviet Union, copying everything from Moscow's five-year economic plans to its approach to mental illness. Soviet authorities, of course, famously used psychiatry to control dissent, spuriously diagnosing thousands of political dissidents as schizophrenics and locking them in asylums. Although China never abused psychiatry to the same extent, the Chinese police still operate some mental hospitals. Occasionally dissidents, including whistleblowers, political critics and adherents of Falun Gong, a spiritual group that meditates through breathing exercises, continue to be dumped in these locked mental facilities (when they aren't being exiled to labor camps).

Critics accuse China of human rights abuses. But Arthur Kleinman, a leading expert on mental illness in China, said his Chinese counterparts have told him that patients brought in by police are immediately discharged if no mental illness is diagnosed. "There is no systematic abuse by the state," Kleinman, a professor of medical anthropology and psychiatry at Harvard University, told *The New York Times*. Tian Zu'en, chief of forensic psychiatry at Beijing's Anding Psychiatric Hospital, agreed. "Our biggest problem is not that normal people are diagnosed as mentally ill, but that ill people are not getting the evaluation and treatment they need."

In Maoist China, being miserable in the workers' paradise was a sin against socialism. In much the way melancholics in medieval Europe were viewed as lacking in God's grace, depressed people in Communist China were suspected of rejecting the socialist dream. Suicide was deemed the ultimate betrayal of the Communist Party and bereaved families received no sympathy.

After Beijing abandoned the Soviet model in the late 1950s, its treatment of mental illness actually worsened, especially in 1966 when Chairman

Mao unleashed the decade of turmoil known as the Cultural Revolution. The Institute of Mental Health in Beijing was shuttered. Psychiatry was classified as a Western bourgeois affectation and pushed to the lowest rung on the medical hierarchy.

At the same time, the Cultural Revolution created a dire need for mental-health professionals. Roiled by successive, increasingly extremist political campaigns, daily life in China became intolerably stressful. Even discussing politics around the dinner table, an important way to let off steam elsewhere, was risky because children, spouses, siblings, friends, neighbors and comrades were encouraged to betray one another, and did. In *Wild Swans*, Jung Chang's best-selling memoir of the Cultural Revolution, she describes her father's nervous breakdown. A top communist official, he disintegrated after his own party turned on him. He remained on tranquilizers, and was in and out of hospitals for the rest of his life.

My husband, Norman, was twenty-two in 1966 when he left New York City for Beijing to study Chinese. At first he thought he had landed in the midst of a civil war. "It looked like Dresden after World War II," he said, describing how rebel factions at the Institute of Industry had used catapults to demolish campus buildings. Later, he biked past a man carrying a samurai sword, "not like it was a souvenir." In 1969, Norman stumbled across two suicide scenes. One man had hanged himself from a tree outside a factory. Another man had flung himself into an irrigation canal.

To Norman, China during the Cultural Revolution gave new meaning to the expression "toxic workplace." In 1970, some staff members at the Foreign Languages Press beat to death half-a-dozen coworkers, and then threw them out the office windows to make it look like they had committed suicide. A few months later, Norman began working there as a translator, and was astounded to find the murderers blithely coming to work as if nothing had happened.

In the apartment building where he lived, Norman became friendly with a Chinese family. He later heard that the mother had attempted suicide after being persecuted by her comrades. "She was a committed communist who had sacrificed everything for the Party. People like her had stood up to much worse trauma on the battlefield, had been captured by the Japanese and put in prison. But what got her was the betrayal by her own."

Norman told me this while I was recovering from my own breakdown. He was pointing my attention toward betrayal as a trigger for depression. Indeed, I believe I could have withstood the hate email, the denunciation by parliament and the death threat, even those goddamn couriered letters from my employer. But what got me in the end, the trigger, was the treatment by *my* comrades—my editors and colleagues, especially in the Montreal bureau, but also the newsroom, who (as I perceived it) abandoned me. In reality, most of them did not have a clue what had happened to me.

Today, after decades of political upheaval, China has a severe shortage of psychiatrists. In a population of 1.3 billion, only 13,000 doctors work in mental health, and only 4,000 of these are psychiatrists. A comparable ratio in New York City would mean just twenty-five shrinks for all five boroughs. Yet as China's economy continues to grow, the Chinese are suffering from the same Go-West-young-man stressors as Americans once did. In the last decade, newfound individualism, unbridled capitalism and unprecedented urban migration have worsened rates of mental illness in China. In various studies conducted between 1982 and 2004, between 1 and 9 percent of Chinese adults reported having a mental disorder. But by 2009, 17 percent of 63,000 Chinese adults reported suffering from a mental disorder. Of those with a diagnosable mental illness, only 5 percent had ever seen a mental-health professional, according to one study that was partly financed by the World Health Organization.

When I arrived in Beijing in 1972 in the midst of the Cultural Revolution, I never heard anyone use the word "depression." Instead, an astonishing number of people would tell me that they suffered from *shenjing shuairuo*, "nervous exhaustion." Many complained of mysterious backaches, headaches, insomnia, lack of energy and loss of appetite, apparently somatizing depression (that is, producing physical symptoms with no apparent organic cause) the way sufferers did in other parts of Asia, including India, Indonesia and Japan. Today the Chinese call depression by its actual name, *yiyu zheng*, literally "the pathology of stress and anxiety." Many, including some of my classmates from Peking University, have begun talking openly about the illness. A prominent television news anchor in Beijing recently revealed, to widespread sympathy, that he suffers from depression.

Some critics call this the Americanization of mental illness. The West has exported a "symptom repertoire," says Ethan Watters, author of *Crazy Like Us: The Globalization of the American Psyche*. He writes that "a handful of mental-health disorders—depression, post-traumatic stress disorder and anorexia among them—now appear to be spreading across cultures with the speed of contagious diseases."

Watters and others point to intensive overseas marketing by Western pharmaceutical companies. They note that the *DSM-IV* has become the standard psychiatric reference throughout the world. They also believe that the attention the West pays to depression might be encouraging its prevalence in other cultures.

I disagree. Depression isn't a uniquely American illness. It transcends national borders, cultures and languages. It strikes people anywhere, everywhere and anytime, whether they know about the symptoms of the disease or not. Ignorance about depression is pervasive, no matter what country you live in. When I was first afflicted by it, I just thought I needed a rest. My inability to write, however, terrified me. Writing was my life, my livelihood, my identity. I would sit at my computer and keep trying. I could type fast enough, but the sentences were disorganized and did not make sense.

I had no idea my predicament was typical. Andrew Solomon had been unable to write during his three bouts with depression. William Styron had the same experience. "I could no longer concentrate during those afternoon hours which for years had been my working time and the act of writing itself, becoming more and more difficult and exhausting, stalled, then finally ceased." Styron considered killing himself. He was stymied, he said, only because he could not write a suicide note.

I began to understand two incidents I had witnessed in the newsroom. A fellow reporter, a business writer, had been hospitalized for depression. He came back a few months later, gaunt and trembling. When I asked how he was doing, he told me that he couldn't write, but management had insisted he get back to work. He quit soon after. More recently, an editor had suffered from anxiety attacks over stresses in her family life. Like the business writer, the editor had also been ordered back prematurely. She worked partial days, which editors can do because others can step in to handle the workflow. Subsequently, however, she had had two serious relapses.

With my own return-to-work order looming, my union kept hoping the problem would go away. Despite what you hear about labor militancy, my union did not want to strain its relations with management. "Please, please, tell me you're better and can go back to work," the union chairperson beseeched me over the phone. What was I suppose to say to that? It felt humiliating to repeat, "I'm sick," over and over. I became almost eager for symptoms. When I couldn't sleep, I felt a bit relieved. It meant I wasn't lying.

Unfortunately, Manulife was refusing to talk to Dr. Au. My union tried to help by requesting her clinical notes and a detailed report. Dr. Au complied and the union quickly delivered both documents to Manulife. I held my breath. I hoped my intervention specialist would agree that I was sick.

CHAPTER 11

A Darker Shade of Blue

In 1990 I was in Hong Kong, hugely pregnant and writing a feature story late one night, when my contractions began. At the time my life revolved around deadlines—and Ben's wasn't for three more weeks—so I ignored the spasms. I finished my story, transmitted it to Toronto and phoned my editor to make sure it got through the ether. Then I dashed to the hospital.

Norman was in Beijing, a three-hour flight away. My labor lasted sixteen hours, enabling him to board a plane the next morning and arrive at the hospital with ten minutes to spare. We were ecstatic when Ben arrived, a wrinkled perfection of tiny fists and downy black hair.

One day later, I was shocked by how blue I felt. I burst into tears for no apparent reason. I refused to take congratulatory calls from friends overseas. I turned away from the lavish flower arrangements sent by the *Globe* and others. Instead of marveling at how lucky I was to have a beautiful baby boy, I saw only reasons to be sad. At five pounds, twelve ounces, Ben was borderline underweight. He had a touch of jaundice. He also had an enzyme deficiency—glucose-6-phosphate dehydrogenase. I had no idea what G6PD was, but when the doctor gave me the news, I burst into tears. After I calmed down, I discovered it meant Ben would become anemic if he ate fava beans or was exposed to mothballs—hardly an epic tragedy.

A couple of weeks later, the blues vanished as quickly as they had come. Like my mother, I had not discussed how I felt with anyone, including my husband or my obstetrician. Only later it occurred to me that I had had a low-grade postpartum depression. When Sam was born three years later, I was prepared and wary. He, too, had a bit of jaundice and he also tested positive for the same enzyme deficiency. But this time around, I didn't shed a single tear. None of this bothered me. I felt just fine.

That earlier experience with postpartum depression, and the later experience without it, gave me insight into how random and unpredictable the blues can be. It also showed me how an internal chemical change can precipitate sadness. A depressive episode is often sparked by a so-called "kindling event"—chronic or severe pain, a stroke, heart attack, general anesthesia, major surgery. It can also be triggered by a major loss—of a person dear to you, of a role, of your image, especially when it involves humiliation or a sense of being trapped.

Paradoxically, even a happy event like the birth of a healthy child can precipitate depression. Other wonderful moments such as getting married, winning a major promotion, being accepted by Harvard Medical School—anything significant enough to roil your internal chemistry—are as likely to kindle depression as a loss. It's as if the gods are laughing at us.

Let me be specific. The gods are mostly laughing at women.

We are twice as likely as men to suffer from depression, even though men are four times as likely to commit suicide. By this I mean unipolar depression, the kind that hit me. In contrast, bipolar or manic depression, strikes equal numbers of men and women. Bipolar women still have more depressive *episodes* than do bipolar men. No one knows why. Scientists do know that the gender gap for unipolar depression sets in at puberty.

Women are more willing to seek help for depression while men try to tough it out. But even when controlling for a reporting bias, researchers still found women suffer major depression twice as often as men do. For instance, twice as many psychotropic drugs are prescribed for women as for men in British Columbia, according to PharmaNet, an electronic network that tracks prescriptions in that province.

Why are women so susceptible? Consciousness remains a mystery, but one hypothesis blames hormones and biochemistry, specifically shifting estrogen levels at childbirth and menopause. After all, women get every kind of depression men get, *plus* postpartum, premenstrual and menopausal blues. And they synthesize serotonin only two-thirds as fast as men do.

Another hypothesis points to that ruinous ruminative cycle. Cognitive psychologists note that women are less likely to grab a semiautomatic and storm the newsroom, blowing everyone to bits. Instead, they are more likely to ruminate. When they are upset, they tend to process their feelings by thinking and thinking and thinking, which only deepen their feelings of gloom. In contrast, men are more likely to express their problems through violence and substance abuse. They are more likely to "go and do something—exercise, use power tools, get drunk, start a war," writes Robert Sapolsky, the neurobiologist who studies stress.

Yet another theory is that female depression is an entirely sane reaction to living in a male-dominated world. Statistically, women are more likely than men to be poor, disenfranchised, uneducated, unemployed or fired. They are much more likely to be sexually abused as children or later abused by a partner or spouse. The social impact of aging also affects women more harshly than men. More men date younger women than older women date younger men. More women than men undergo painful facelifts (although men are quickly catching up). More male actors get juicy roles past the age of thirty, Meryl Streep being an exception that proves the rule.

If you give any credence to the oppression theory, consider that gays are more likely to be rejected by their families, suffer from discrimination in housing and employment and experience public humiliation. In a homophobic world, they often feel compelled to live a lie, which is corrosive to self-esteem. Given all this, gays should have significantly higher rates of depression and suicide than heterosexuals have. And they do.

If you give weight to the rumination theory, then men should be the ones who go postal, commit school shootings and murder their families. And they do. In China, where guns are difficult to obtain, a series of seven mass stabbings and cleaver and hammer attacks left at least twenty-one dead and ninety injured in 2010. In each case, the perpetrator was male and the victims were mostly elementary school children.

A famous study of school shooters by the U.S. Secret Service found that all the killers were male and all had experienced a significant loss, grievance or sense of failure that led them to commit suicide in the most vengeful way possible. The three shooters at Dawson College and Columbine High School, for instance, all reported depression toward the end of their lives. The Dawson commission of inquiry found that Kimveer Gill had visited a clinic complaining of suicidal thoughts a few months before his rampage. He had taken antidepressants, but quit when they had little effect. His mother said that in the weeks before the shootings, he had been sleeping a lot and drinking heavily, mostly Jack Daniel's whiskey. She had never seen him sadder, but neither she nor anyone else understood that he was sick.

"I'd ask him if anything was wrong, and he said, 'No, nothing'," Parvinder Gill told reporters. "He was twenty-five, what was I supposed to do? I never even thought to take away the guns because he just wasn't like that. He never hurt anyone."

Eric Harris and Dylan Klebold killed fifteen people and wounded twenty-three more at Columbine before committing suicide. The report by a review commission stated that Harris had been taking antidepressants. His autopsy results revealed a therapeutic level of the antidepressant drug Luvox. The same report included this entry from Klebold's journal: "I swear—like I'm an outcast, and everyone is conspiring against me ... Fact: People are so unaware ... well, ignorance is bliss I guess ... that would explain my depression."

Gill and Harris received medical attention, though clearly not enough.

Researchers estimate that only half of American adults who have major depression seek help of any kind, even from a priest. That proportion is reflected consistently throughout most of the developed world. In the United States alone 17 million people go untreated for depression. In Britain, the half that seeks help usually goes to family doctors, where only a minority will be properly diagnosed and fewer still will receive appropriate treatment.

The vast majority of depressives, of course, will not go on the rampage. Those who embark on a shooting spree are not only depressed, they are severely psychotic and out of touch with reality. They are also clinically narcissistic, so pathologically self-focused that they fail to consider the consequences of their actions on others. Despite garnering intense media attention, these murderous sprees are rare enough to be considered psychiatric curiosities. Psychiatrists aren't sure what prompts school shooters to commit suicide against a tableau of mass murder. What is clear is the toll.

In 2010, a landmark three-year study of the impact of school shootings showed that nearly one third of bystanders suffered psychological damage, including post-traumatic stress, substance abuse, major depression or a social phobia as a direct result of what they had experienced. The study, funded by the Quebec government in the wake of the Dawson College shootings, is the first to examine the psychological impact of such an event. Researchers at the McGill University Health Centre and Louis-H. Lafontaine Hospital, a psychiatric hospital in Montreal, interviewed nearly one thousand students and staff at Dawson College. The study found they suffered psychological damage at a rate two to three times higher than that of the general population, and that the trauma increased with proximity to the shooting. Those who witnessed the actual attack, heard the shots or hid in an office or classroom were three or four times more likely to develop a psychiatric disorder, according to Warren Steiner, a member of the research team. The study noted that their problems extended well beyond the eight-month period for which Dawson College provided counseling service. Those with pre-existing disorders reported feeling the effects for up to eighteen months.

From the 1999 rampage at Columbine High School to the publication of the Dawson College study in 2010, there have been at least sixty school shootings. Imagine the pain felt by each survivor; the members of each victim's family; the trauma experienced by police officers, paramedics and emergency personnel who rushed to the scene and by all the medical workers who later treated the dying and the wounded; the anguish of the murderer's own family. And then imagine the emotional shock waves spreading out, engulfing countless more families and friends.

I wasn't even present when Kimveer Gill stormed into the college. Yet the event overwhelmed me, changed my life and impacted those around me.

In evolutionary terms, cortisol was originally helpful. Back when our ancestors encountered a saber-toothed tiger, cortisol, a "fight-or-flight" hormone like adrenalin, was the magic system-override. To deploy every resource to cope with an immediate threat, cortisol would prevent our bodies from momentarily replenishing the essential nutrients required to rebuild muscles, joints, nerves and brain circuits. It would interrupt work of the digestive system and halt production of immunoglobulin A, an antibody required by the immune system to fight colds and the flu. Robert Sapolsky, author of *Why Zebras Don't Get Ulcers*, notes that cortisol mobilizes energy in thigh muscles, increases blood pressure and turns off everything that isn't essential to short-term survival, including digestion, growth and reproduction.

Those pre-historic folks whose systems failed to flood with cortisol presumably shrugged at the tiger, and were then eaten. In evolutionary terms, they were losers because, well, they were dead and had no further chance of passing on their genes. The folks whose bodies flooded with the stress hormone went into fight-or-flight mode and survived, increasing the odds that they would pass on their genes. In evolutionary terms, they were winners.

The system worked well, chemically speaking, in prehistoric times. Wrestling a wild animal or running for your life are intense physical activities that consume glucose and burn off excessive cortisol. Unfortunately, stressors in the modern world don't usually include tigers, unless you happen to work at a zoo. Instead, we struggle with chronic problems such as financial worries, traffic jams, flight delays, dysfunctional families, street crime and toxic workplaces. Nevertheless these same primeval juices continue to flood the body, even though we are no longer able to burn off the stress hormone. (You *can* run screaming from a predatory manager, but you'll probably end up with a note in your personnel file.)

For the common office primate, a life spent awash in cortisol is toxic. Cortisol can stun the heart muscle, potentially leading to a heart attack. Other devastating health consequences include adult-onset diabetes, high blood pressure, heart disease, stroke and various gastrointestinal disorders, including stomachaches, gastroenteritis, colitis and ulcers.

Sustained stress can also impair learning, memory and judgment, partly because rumination hijacks consciousness, leaving less brainpower for memory and executive function.

"Getting tense in the face of a threat was adaptive for our ancestors," writes Daniel J. Levitin, a researcher at McGill University. "It is maladaptive for us when those stressors are long-term, chronic and don't require an acute physical response."

Cortisol is released by all kinds of stressors, from the death of a loved one to a surprise birthday party. The more of it released during shock or stress, the more likely depression will occur. Prolonged stress can even lead to brain lesions. The latest research on brain elasticity shows that stress and depression actually realign the neurons, causing a relapse even without a major triggering event. And unfortunately, stress and depression also destroy the very neurons that should regulate cortisol levels—long after the stress is resolved.

Robert Sapolsky, who spent three decades studying African baboons in the wild, says they make useful research models. Like humans, baboons in the Serengeti don't have real predators. And baboons need toil only three hours a day for their calories, which gives them about nine leisure hours daily to psychologically torment other baboons in their troop. Like unhealthy people, unhealthy baboons have elevated resting levels of stress hormones, Sapolsky discovered. "They're just like us. They're not getting done in by predators and famines; they're getting done in by each other," he writes. "Primates are super smart and organized just enough to devote their free time to being miserable to each other and stressing each other out."

Ever since my Dawson feature story was published, I felt as though I were fleeing tigers day and night. With my cortisol levels persistently elevated, my neck and shoulder muscles were always tense. I was so stiff I could barely turn my head and when I did, I heard tiny, crackling noises.

Now when I think back to the last year of my mother's life, I realize that the stressors had piled up for her until she succumbed to depression. A decade earlier, she had been diagnosed with heart disease, an early sign of stress. Then she had heart surgery, another precipitator of depression. She had fought back from that, but a few years later, there was another kindling event, a stroke that left her paralyzed on one side and unable to speak. Working doggedly with physiotherapists, she tossed basketballs from her wheelchair and forced herself to walk a few feet every day. She worked through stacks of flashcards with pictures of fruits and vegetables, struggling to speak the right words: "celery," "potato," "apple," "mushroom."

Mom heroically regained almost all her mobility and speech. Then a post-stroke MRI scan found cancer. She had another major operation under general anesthetic to remove most of one lung, another kindling event. She suffered intense post-operative pain, yet another kindling event. It was all too much. When her doctor prescribed antidepressants, I encouraged her to take them, but I never discussed how she was feeling. I instinctively shied away from talking about depression (even though I had no problem asking difficult questions about her last wishes).

I watched helplessly as Mom lost her appetite. When I visited her in Montreal, I cooked her favorite Chinese dish, steamed rice with ginger-scallion chicken. I tried to entice her with delicate portions, artfully arranged on her best china. She took a bite and shook her head. Although she valiantly forced down can after can of strawberry, chocolate and vanilla Ensure, a calorie-rich proprietary drink, she still lost weight. Mom lingered for two hard years. At her death, she weighed just sixty-five pounds.

I didn't fully understand how stress impacts metabolism until I experienced depression myself. As we've seen, in pre-historic times the stress hormone suppressed your appetite to make your getaway as efficient as possible. You temporarily stopped digesting food and storing up energy. You ran for your life on *stored* energy. Then, after you escaped the saber-toothed tiger, your adrenal gland released glucocorticoids to stimulate your appetite so that you could start replenishing your now-depleted stores of energy.

In the modern world, one third of people lose their appetite when stressed. The other two thirds eat *more* than normal. Which group you fall into "is accomplished through some endocrinology that is initially fairly confusing, but is actually really elegant," writes Sapolsky. When stressed, lab rats are like humans: they split into those that eat more and those that eat less. And like lab rats, humans will gain or lose weight depending on the type and pattern of stressors.

In both mammals, the hypothalamus sends out an appetite inhibitor called corticotropin-releasing hormone in the first few seconds of a stressful event. If the stressor lasts for days, humans and rats will lose their appetites—and lose weight. But if the stressor is intermittent, as soon as the situation improves, the *appetite-inhibiting* corticotropin-releasing hormone will be followed by the release of *appetite-stimulating* glucocorticoids. Your body thinks you've just dashed across the savannah and now that the stressor/threat has passed, you need to replenish your stores of energy. You haven't actually dashed across the savannah, but you still feel hungry and tend to overeat. You gain weight.

In the modern world, intermittent stressors are unavoidable (and usually involve sedentary behavior). They may include your monthly Visa bill, rush-hour traffic, the boss yelling at you at the Monday morning departmental meeting. The bad news for those who face these intermittent stressors is that glucocorticoids don't merely stimulate appetite. They stimulate it *preferentially* for starchy, sweet and fatty foods. That is why intermittently stressed-out people mindlessly nosh throughout the day on comfort foods like French fries, cookies and cupcakes.

It isn't fair. On top of all your problems, you also gain weight.

In my case, the ongoing strife with my employer lasted weeks and months, with brand-new triggers piling on, and no end in sight. Excess cortisol inundated my system, preparing me for never-ending fight or flight, shutting down my digestive system, preventing me from absorbing nutrients. Meanwhile my hypothalamus thought I was stuck in the initial run-from-the-tiger phase and it kept secreting corticotropin-releasing hormone, suppressing my appetite. I never got to the glucocorticoid donut-eating stage.

When Dr. Au noticed my weight was dropping, she urged me to eat. I tried, and I'm sure some food got down. But until I read Sapolsky, I didn't understand how I could eat fries, donuts and whipped cream *and* still lose weight. Like Mom, who in the final months of her life couldn't see any end to her problems either, I lost weight steadily. My digestive system had shut down. I was experiencing the adult version of "failure to thrive," the syndrome in which an infant loses weight because of a genetic metabolism problem or because the mother is absent, incompetent or suffering from postpartum depression.

In my case, I had rarely lost weight before. For two decades, despite two pregnancies and incipient middle age, my weight had held steady at around 127 pounds, just about right for my height. Then in two months I lost 17 pounds. It didn't seem like a lot, but it was 13 percent of my body weight. Dr. Au was concerned enough that she began weighing me every week. My wedding ring felt loose, my shoes seemed too big and my jeans slipped down my hips. I dropped four clothes sizes, to a size two. If I lost any more weight, I'd have to shop in the children's section. But—and I admit this is incredibly superficial—my weight loss was the unmentionable silver lining of depression. I was suddenly svelte. As a middle-aged mother of two, I never expected to have a flat stomach again. Losing so much weight, however, wasn't really healthy. Some friends said I looked gaunt. I was definitely weak. I struggled to open doors or a jar of mayonnaise. At night

I was grinding my teeth so badly that I chipped two upper molars.

The solution to my troubles with management—not the cure for my illness—seemed blindingly obvious. I could have gone back into the office and made like I was working. After all, writing feature stories is an elusive enterprise: a single piece sometimes takes many days to produce. But I had seen what happened to my two colleagues who had returned to work prematurely. And Dr. Au had warned me that returning to the office early could make me even sicker.

That December the company issued me a total of two back-to-work orders. Then it hired outside lawyers to fight my disability claim, my first ever. I was terrified. But somewhere between the ultimatums and the looming legal fight, I made a decision. I was sick, and I had a right to be sick. If the whole world kept caving to employers, we would never recognize depression as a true illness. When I look back now, I see this was a turning point. For the first time, I stopped wavering about whether or not I was sick.

Depression does not transform you into someone else. It sits, like a cloud, over your original personality. If you are normally stubborn and fierce about your rights, you don't become a doormat just because you are depressed. I may have been fragile and forgetful, prone to tears and lacking in self-esteem. But I remained, for better or worse, as pig-headed and bloody-minded as before. I abhorred the company's insinuation that I was lying about my illness.

At my next appointment, Dr. Au repeated her opinion: I wasn't well enough to return to work. I cried, tears of relief and despair. At least it meant I wasn't shirking my duties. Yet it also meant I was still sick. I told my doctor I was dying to leave town again. I didn't understand why I was so desperate to get away from my situation. Instinctively I needed to put as much physical distance between my tormenters (as I saw them) and myself. In hindsight I realize I was fleeing the metaphorical tigers.

Five months earlier I had signed on to accompany Sam's hockey team to Finland and Sweden over the Christmas break. Now I asked whether I should I go or not. "You should go," Dr. Au said. "It will be good for you to get away. You need to focus on your family. Don't talk about your situation. It will be a complete break."

I exhaled. Perhaps I'd return home restored and ready to write.

Dr. Au once again urged me to start taking antidepressants. She warned they could take from four to eight weeks to kick in. I had never opened the free starter kit of Effexor she had given me. Instead, like everyone else these days, I had gone on the Internet to check the drug. I found scary side effects, including nausea, dizziness, nervousness, constipation, sweating, dry mouth, loss of appetite and, confusingly, sleepiness *and* insomnia, not to mention unspecified sexual side effects. "All patients should be watched for becoming agitated, irritable, hostile, aggressive, impulsive, restless, or anxious," a website revealed. It added that antidepressants could worsen depression to the point of making the patient suicidal.

I was too scared to start Effexor when I was far away from Dr. Au. I told her I would wait until after the hockey trip. I still kept hoping I would recover without meds. To me antidepressants were an acknowledgment of weakness, a failure of will. At that point I still didn't comprehend that my shame was the legacy of centuries of stigma. But that is why everyone congratulates you when they hear you have weaned yourself off antidepressants. The implication: there's even something wrong with taking the medicine for this illness.

Dr. Au changed her tack. "Maybe you should see a psychiatrist," she said. I shook my head, too upset to speak. A psychiatrist treats crazy people. I wasn't crazy. There was nothing really wrong with me. When I started to weep again, Dr. Au dropped the subject and wrote me another sick note.

Later that day, one of the hockey dads stopped by my home to pick up the final payment for the Scandinavian trip. I was writing out the check when he said, with some embarrassment, that he had to ask me something. "Some of the parents wanted to know if you could promise not to write about the trip." In my depressed state, I was instantly and deeply offended. To me it seemed that now the hockey parents wanted to silence me, too. Stubbornly, I refused to promise anything, but told the dad the truth, that I had no intention of writing about the trip. I didn't tell him the whole truth: I was no longer able to write at all.

I duly sent Dr. Au's latest sick note to the HR department. The union's lawyer advised me not to go to work until I recovered, and to let the second and final company-imposed deadline pass. On December 13, the *Globe* stopped my sick pay and all my benefits. When a couriered letter arrived announcing the stoppage, I sobbed until my eyes were swollen. I stuck a little blue Ativan pill under my tongue. The tears stopped.

Glumly I considered my prospects. For the first time in my working life, I would be without a paycheck. With Norman still jobless, how would we pay for groceries? I wrote out a chronological list of worst-case scenarios. At the bottom of my list, I wrote: "Fired." I stared at the word. It couldn't happen. Or could it? And would I have the courage to stick it out to the end?

Twelve days before Christmas, another letter arrived by courier. It was a demand for payment for my old notes from the maid series. Several months before Dawson I had taken a short, unpaid leave to start writing a book on the minimum wage. Exactly how much I was now supposed to cough up for used notes was never made clear. Nevertheless I refused. Have I mentioned I'm pig-headed? As far as I knew, no one at the newspaper had ever been asked to pay for used notes. The letter from management ordered me to come to terms "within a week." Otherwise, the deputy editor warned, she would contact my book publisher to stop publication. I cried again, this time out of fear, frustration and anger, and popped another tranquilizer.

Next the vice-president of human resources telephoned. She said that by writing Dr. Au's name on the disclosure form, I had invalidated it. Therefore Manulife couldn't talk to Dr. Au. No matter that Manulife had already received her notes and detailed report, thanks to the union's intervention. The vice-president of human resources said the insurer could not and would not look at the documents.

Allow me to take a moment here, with the benefit of hindsight, to discuss how a good human resources department might have handled this. Obviously, they can't *diagnose* depression, but spotting troubled employees is a crucial business skill, considering that almost three in ten employees will suffer from mental health problems in any given year, and that the average length of time off work in each instance is thirty days.

So, first of all, human resources staff should be educated about the common symptoms. These include any abrupt changes in behavior at work, such as suddenly being unable to cope with assignments, apparent distraction, crying jags, loss of motivation or uncharacteristic absenteeism. They should also understand that an occasional blip of this kind is not depression—only when the signs persist longer than two weeks.

Of course, depression can be caused either by a workplace or personal issue or by a chemical imbalance. Human resources staff should try to find a moment to talk privately but informally with the employee. If they establish the problem is either personal or a chronic chemical one, they can point the person to their doctor or to counseling and other services. If the issue is work-related, then human resources has the added responsibility of providing temporary relief from the stressor and seeking a long-term remedy.

The most important goal for a good human resources department is to create a work culture that is sensitive to mental illness. In doing so, they will help eradicate some of the stigma and reduce pressure on the sick employee, possibly resulting in shorter and fewer absences. But if the human resources department takes an aggressive stance—suggesting, for instance, that the employee is a liar and a malingerer, and handles the symptoms from an absenteeism and performance perspective—the company may end up sabotaging its own best interests. It will almost surely incur numerous additional costs, including buy-outs or settlements, legal fees and excessive management time, not to mention low employee morale as others watch from the sidelines.

From my perspective as an employee, the stress was unremitting. Perhaps I would have recovered faster with some sympathy and understanding. Instead it seemed as though every time I came up for air, someone smashed me on the head. I felt like one of the pop-up furry mammals in that silly arcade game, Whac-a-Mole. I spiraled downward. I became as paranoid as I had been while working in China, where the secret police often tailed me and people I interviewed were sometimes detained. I told Norman I feared someone might break into our house and steal my maid notebooks. Perhaps I should stash a set with a friend? He said nothing, but he quietly went to Kinko's to photocopy every page.

Just when I was sure I could sink no lower, my older brother announced the closure of the family business. The restaurant had been struggling in a difficult economy and the boycott launched by Le Québécois website might have been the death knell. "Bill Wong's, one of Montreal's landmark restaurants, is closing its doors next month," the Gazette reported on December 15, 2006. "The eatery on Décarie Blvd. just north of Jean Talon St., a fixture among Chinese restaurants since it opened in 1963, will cease to exist after Jan. 7."

Cease to exist. I wept again. I was only eleven and so proud when Dad opened Bill Wong's, the biggest Chinese restaurant in what was then Canada's biggest city. Bill Wong's had two main-floor dining rooms, several upstairs banquet rooms, two bars, a disco-dance floor and a Japanese teppanyaki steak house. Dad couldn't cook to save his life, but he was a smart businessman. With his engineering background, he designed an open-ended egg roll that customers loved because it could be stuffed with extra cabbage and spicy shredded pork.

In the 1950s, he had been the first Montrealer to open a Chinese restaurant outside Chinatown, catering to those too timid to venture there. He quickly opened several more. He began offering free delivery, at a time when the only food ordered over the phone in the city was barbecue chicken. In the early 1960s, he thought he could do better than the ubiquitous "dinner for two" and launched the first all-you-can-eat Chinese buffet, an innovation quickly copied by Chinese restaurants throughout North America and beyond. For forty-three years, his flagship restaurant employed Quebeckers, Japanese-Canadians and immigrants from China, Hong Kong, Vietnam, Sri Lanka and Greece.

Three months earlier when I set out to report the rampage at Dawson College, I never anticipated that one casualty might be my family's business. Not only had I destroyed my father's legacy, I ruined my relationship with my brother Earl, who had managed the flagship restaurant and now lost his livelihood. Earl and I had never been close. At this point we became completely estranged.

I phoned my father and tried to apologize.

"It's okay," Dad said. "Never mind."

No one at the *Globe* ever acknowledged my family's loss.

The balance in my checking account steadily dwindled. Every time I bought something, I felt scared. Four friends separately offered financial help, which I declined. My sister, ever the accountant, calmed me down and reminded me I had investments.

That Christmas, I didn't feel much like celebrating but I tried for a semblance of normalcy. We bought our usual fresh-cut spruce tree from IKEA for twenty dollars and decorated it with sequined balls and my collection of Mao buttons. Norman usually confines his gift giving to small items I circle in a gardening catalogue, but this year, I didn't have the energy. To my utter astonishment, he went to Home Depot and bought me a new stove (after first prudently clearing the model with me). I'd been whining for years about how annoyingly weak our old one was for searing or stir-frying. The wonderful white-enameled General Electric stove had a 17,500-BTU super burner, a nifty warming drawer and a fifth burner that could be converted to a grill. Some people might think this gift was unromantic but I felt happy for the first time in weeks. To me, the stove was elemental—a symbol of warmth, food and security—everything I felt had been taken away from me.

Norman's gift reminded me that we had a hearth and home together. Depression can tear some families asunder. The lucky ones get stronger. My husband was always there in the background, protective of me and observant. When he told me how betrayed his Beijing neighbor had felt during the Cultural Revolution, I felt that he really understood me. He could reflect back to me what I was unable at the time to do for myself. He was supportive, staunch and steadfast, for better and for worse, for richer, for poorer, in sickness and in health.

CHAPTER 12

The Music Cure

I celebrated Christmas with fingers crossed in hopes of a miracle. Then, in fight-or-flight mode, I jumped on a plane for Helsinki for another dose of the geographic cure. The more my writing failed me, the more I fell back on my motherhood role. I was looking forward to two whole weeks with Sam. I didn't understand that depression reverses roles and flips relationships inside out. I was the mother, but increasingly I looked to my thirteen-year-old son to mother me. I had become narcissistically needy, pathologically clingy.

In a daze, I got on and off buses in small towns with names such as Lohja, Sandviken and Leksand. I checked into quaint hotels with gingerbread trim and Spartan dorm rooms at rural sports institutes. I ate breakfast by candlelight and watched hockey game after hockey game. I must have been pretty far gone to expect a cure for depression in a land where the sun sets by early afternoon. Everything made me cry: the bare trees dusted with snow, the endless bus rides, even standing at attention for a scratchy, pregame rendition of "O Canada."

I was a hockey mom having a nervous breakdown. At a game in Sweden, I began to weep in earnest. Our team was getting slaughtered: nine goals against us in the first five *minutes*. Sam's co-goalie had been in net, but now my son was about to take his place. Suddenly, through a blur of tears, I watched the coaches confer. Soon half the Swedish team was donning Canadian jerseys and half the Canadian team was donning Swedish jerseys. The mixed teams played happily together, each thrilled to be wearing the others' colors. Like an idiot, I cried even harder.

I remained deeply depressed, but at least the geographic cure was diverting. I steamed myself hot pink in a Finnish sauna, and then ran barefoot and naked through darkness and gale-force winds down a stony path and a wooden staircase to the frozen dock. I dipped a toe in the slushy lake, which was one degree away from forming ice. I gasped in shock. Gritting my teeth, I forced myself in until the water reached my armpits. I thought I would have a heart attack. Instantly I hauled myself out and raced back, footprints freezing on the dock, up the staircase and up the stony path, to the sauna.

Later, I suggested to a Finnish parent that the custom seemed a tad extreme. "You jumped in the lake?" she said, surprised. "We only do that in the summer."

Sam was a newcomer on the team and by extension I was, too. A couple of the dads were friendly, and one mom was especially kind, so kind that I disregarded Dr. Au's advice and confided in her. Mostly, though, I remember the pain of exclusion. I felt constantly rebuffed. Each day, I forced myself to approach tables occupied by other parents, only to discover the seats were saved for someone else. I felt like weeping as I sat alone at meals. I was as insecure and unhappy as a pimply adolescent who had been transferred to a new high school.

Were the others afraid I would quote them? Were they angry I wouldn't guarantee not to write about the trip? Had they noticed my twitching eye and feared I was an axe murderer? I was still splitting into two: the depressed person devastated by rejection and the professional observer who noted how far I had strayed from my usually confident self.

I noticed I had become hypersensitive to slights, or perceived slights. From one mother, I learned the hard way that depressed people attract bullies. On the first day of the trip, she asked if her son could borrow Sam's hockey socks. Her son had forgotten to pack his and the coach was threatening to bench him for the uniform infraction. I so desperately wanted to make friends, I eagerly agreed—without even consulting my son. (I reasoned that, as Sam was a goalie, the coach wouldn't notice if he wasn't wearing regulation socks under his thigh-high leg pads. But still, I should have asked Sam.)

The woman must have sensed my neediness, my aura of hopelessness. When I later took a seat beside her on the bus, she scowled and made it clear she preferred that I sit elsewhere. On another occasion, when I set down my backpack on the seat beside her at a hockey arena, she frowned.

"Can you move that? It bothers me."

My old self would have told *her* to move her ass because *she* bothered *me*. Instead, I obeyed. I silently picked up the offending bag, and put it on my lap. In doing so, I was overwhelmed with self-loathing. I had become so weak, so full of despair that I had the self-esteem of a tapeworm. I felt utterly worthless.

Mostly I shared a room with Sam. In Sandviken, where the boys were billeted with Swedish families, we parents were randomly paired off at the local hotel. I was pleased, thrilled actually, to discover I would be bunking with one of the more outgoing mothers. Perhaps through her I might break into the hockey-mom clique. But outside the hotel, as I was collecting my suitcase from the storage compartment beneath the bus, "It bothers me" stopped me.

"*I'm* rooming with her," she snapped, snatching the room key from my hand.

The old me would have snatched it right back. The new, damaged, vulnerable me accepted the bullying and tried not to burst into tears. Months later, I learned that both women were having marriage problems. Perhaps they wanted to room with each other for mutual support. In hindsight, I wonder if we were all too much on edge to see one another's pain.

When I read this now, I seem unbelievably pathetic. Did the other parents actually ostracize me? Or did depression distort my view of reality? All I know is that the pain then was as real to me as if I had sliced my arm open with a knife.

In my despair, I glommed onto Sam, quite literally. Photos from the trip show me grinning at the camera—you can always grin, no matter how much you are dying inside—always holding onto Sam, leaning in toward him, gripping his arm. In one, I've got both arms clamped around his shoulder. How oppressive this must have felt to him. But I had suffered too many losses, and I couldn't bear the thought of losing him too. Whenever I couldn't actually see him, at an airport or on the bus or on the street, I would panic and bellow his name as though he were three years old instead of thirteen.

"It was annoying," he recalls now, carefully choosing the strongest word he knows that won't make me cry. "You were always shouting, '*Sam! Sam!*' It was so embarrassing."

I can't believe I did that to my son. I was never like that before. I let him use the stove and oven, supervised, of course, when he was only five. When he was eleven, I encouraged him to travel alone on Toronto's far-flung subway system. But depression blinds you to others' needs. It leaves you no emotional space to consider others, even those you love. You're like a drowning person who can't help clutching the next person, even a loved one, and dragging them down.

At the time, I didn't get how humiliating it was for Sam. But he could see how awful things were for me. He would notice me eating by myself and be torn between consoling his shattered mother and hanging out with his new teammates. He compromised by sitting with me at breakfast when the other boys were still semi-comatose. Unfortunately I would pester him for company at lunch and supper, too.

Sam recalled, "I would always ask, 'Can I *please* just eat with the team?'"

The last night of the trip, he wanted to play ping-pong in the hotel with the others. The healthy me would have encouraged him to bond with his teammates. His happiness would have made me happy. "No," I said, stonily. By then I had given up trying to make friends with the other parents. I was furious with everyone. And I couldn't stand being alone anymore.

"Why can't I?"

"We have a long flight tomorrow," I said, grasping at parental straws. "If you don't get enough sleep, you'll get sick. And school's starting on Monday."

"I can sleep on the flight. Please, can I hang out with everyone?"

"No," I snapped.

And then things got ugly. I wept and raged. I called him selfish and ungrateful. I said I had paid thousands of dollars for the trip at a time when my sick pay had been stopped. (This wasn't true; I had paid for the trip six months earlier.) But my pent-up anger at the way I'd been treated, or thought I'd been treated, erupted. I said I had wasted my time coming to Scandinavia because he had no time for me. I said he didn't care about me. That night I sank to the lowest point of my entire illness. At thirteen, Sam was the mature adult in our relationship. Between sobs, he explained again and again, patiently, without ever once raising his voice, how desperately he was trying to be part of the team. I refused to relent. We cried ourselves to sleep, side by side, in narrow twin beds at a hotel near the Stockholm airport.

"I just wanted to hang out with them," says Sam, two years later, still upset. "Even someone's little sister, who was *nine*, was allowed to stay up."

The next day, exhausted, we flew home from Stockholm via London's Heathrow Airport, arriving in Toronto in the early evening. At the luggage carousel, I heard someone call my name. She was a journalism professor I knew. An instant later, I remembered she was married to Ed Greenspon. And a moment after *that*, I realized my editor-in-chief was standing right beside me.

We had been on the same jumbo jet from London. Bizarrely, we had picked the very same spot to wait for our luggage. Greenspon greeted me curtly, and then turned his back on me. It took all my strength not to bolt. My left eye began twitching. My hands trembled. I felt waves of guilt, as though I'd been caught red-handed gallivanting around the globe (when I should have been lying in bed with a thermometer in my mouth). Panicky thoughts filled my head. *I shouldn't have listened to Dr. Au. How could travel be a legitimate treatment for depression?*

Despite our blowup the previous night, Sam stuck loyally by my side. Eventually my editor-in-chief's suitcases materialized and he left without a word. My jet-lagged teen and I waited some more. Finally the empty carousel shuddered to a halt. British Airways had lost our luggage, the final, absurd twist in a horrible trip.

I held my tears until we arrived home. Sam went into his room without a word and closed the door. Ben listened patiently while I wept and told him about the chance encounter with my boss. He hugged me, stroking my back, as if I were the child. "Nothing's changed," he said gently. "They didn't think you were sick before and they don't think you're sick now."

It was a Sunday. On Monday the editor-in-chief must have told the HR vice-president about the airport encounter because she immediately called the union chairperson to say I shouldn't have been traveling while receiving short-term disability. "Well, it's a good thing she's not receiving any benefits," the union chairperson snapped.

The next day was the final day of business for my father's restaurant. Dad went to visit Bill Wong's one last time. At eighty-six, leaning on his cane, he made his way through the dining rooms and the kitchen, greeting the staff and bidding farewell to customers who had come one last time.

I stayed in Toronto. I felt as though I had precipitated the death of the family business. It was too painful to contemplate being there at the end.

A steady diet of herring and Swedish meatballs had helped me to gain three pounds. Encouraged, I joined a health club but could not keep pace with the aerobics class. Not only was I weak, my brain couldn't follow the instructor's left-foot, right-foot moves. I quit after four sessions.

Music was better. Like the geographic cure, it transported me to another place. Music feeds the soul, a truth the ancients understood. "Music produces a kind of pleasure which human nature cannot do without," Confucius said.

Besides going to as many concerts as I could, I began playing my flute, an instrument I had learned in high school. I had dropped it for years, then briefly joined the North Toronto Community Band, but soon quit, too busy with career and family. A few years later, the band president phoned to say they needed flutes, so I gave it another try. I was terrible, but the other members— there were about forty—didn't kick me out and I gradually improved.

Now that I was sick, I looked forward to our Monday night rehearsals with delight. We practiced a repertoire of marches, jazz, big band, Disney medleys, soft rock and dumbed-down classical music. Each year we would perform several concerts, almost exclusively at retirement homes, where the audiences were suitably captive and hearing-impaired.

As I became more adept, I was invited to play in a woodwind trio with Robert Hall, an oboist, and Holli Verkade, a clarinetist. We would meet weekly in one of our homes for a civilized two-hour practice. It was civilized because Robert, an elderly British gentleman, did not approve of swearing, which Holli and I would otherwise lapse into during particularly difficult passages. It felt wonderfully eighteenth-century to be cocooned in sounds of our own making. And, yes, we also performed at retirement homes.

In the midst of my depression, Lori Scopis, a fellow flautist in the band, invited me to join a flute ensemble. Each Wednesday night, we would struggle through a challenging repertoire of Latin sambas, Handel, Mozart and the blindingly fast "Flight of the Bumblebee" (which in my case should more truthfully be dubbed, "Bumble"). Our conductor, Gennady Gefter, a ginger-haired Russian émigré, was a stern taskmaster, the kind who was livid if we failed to arrive twenty minutes early to warm up. He died a thousand deaths with every incorrect note, sloppy entry or *mezzo piano* that should have been a *pianissimo*. He would berate us for breathing at the wrong moment ("never on a bar line!") or for holding a note a nanosecond too long—or too short. His criticism was withering, and spot on. Once, when I played a note shockingly out-of-tune, he barked, "Don't play! *Just! Don't! Play!*" And all this grief to perform at, yes, retirement homes.

Many flautists quit the ensemble in disgust or out of pure fear, which created a never-ending membership crisis. It's a wonder I didn't walk out too. I was so sensitive to criticism I should have shriveled up, but I stayed because Gennady is a superb teacher. He would explain how to play harmonics, how to hit high notes softly (and *why* we should) and how to use alternate fingering so we could play as fast as, well, a bumblebee. He would show us how to stand, slightly curved at the waist, to maximize lung capacity. He would demonstrate the magic of a particular phrase of music, playing his heart out for us, hoping we'd eventually get it. Sometimes I felt like I never would. But I *am* playing more musically now and recently I realized I am even beginning to play (sometimes) in tune.

I always feel happier after playing music. It turns out I'm not imagining this. Scientists have found that the act of making music increases the brain's dopamine, the so-called "feel-good" hormone. No one is quite sure *why* dopamine floods the brain, but Daniel Levitin, a Montreal-based musician and researcher, has proposed an evolutionary explanation in *The World in Six Songs*. "Our ancestors who were able to communicate with music, and who *enjoyed* musical communication, may well have been at a distinct advantage to ..." defuse tense social situations "... that might otherwise have led to combat and death. What we know for certain is that increases in dopamine lead to elevated mood and help to boost the immune system."

In other words, you not only feel good emotionally when you perform music, but you also feel good *physically* because dopamine also sparks an upsurge of immunoglobulin A, which fights colds, the flu and other infections. Blood tests administered to people right after a singing lesson also show measurably higher levels of oxytocin, the same hormone released during orgasm and breast-feeding, according to a 2003 research paper published in *Integrative Physiological & Behavioral Science*. There are also increases in melatonin, noradrenalin, adrenalin (norepinephrine, epinephrine) and serotonin, all naturally occurring chemicals in the brain that variously affect depression, arousal and mood. "Listening to, and even more so singing or playing, music can alter brain chemistry associated with well-being, stress reduction, and immune system fortitude," Levitin writes.

When she was U.S. secretary of state, Condoleezza Rice would rehearse with two violinists, a violist and a cellist every two weeks in her Watergate apartment. A favorite piece was the Brahms Piano Quintet in F Minor, Opus 34. Asked by *The New York Times* if she found the sessions relaxing, Rice, a classically trained pianist, said, "It's not exactly relaxing if you are struggling to play Brahms, but it is transporting. When you're playing there is only room for Brahms or Shostakovich. It's the time I'm most away from myself and I treasure it."

For me, too, playing music (and trying to stay in tune) is never relaxing, but it *is* transporting. It's the audio equivalent of flight. It doesn't matter whether I am playing the third-flute part of "Swing Low, Sweet Chariot" or a tricky Bach fugue. Musical performance demands a high level of focus, with no time to ruminate about death threats. All you can worry about is whether Maestro Gefter is about to slaughter you instead.

The first days of the New Year passed in a blur. I was still deeply depressed and unable to write. Complicating matters was a pending book leave. Management wanted me to start the unpaid leave, on schedule, on January 1. From their perspective, the earlier I completed the two-month book leave, the earlier I could start producing stories for them again. From my perspective, I couldn't go on a book leave when I couldn't write. Frankly, I couldn't see why management cared so much. They were saving money whether I was on book leave or sick leave: either way they weren't paying me. But the dispute over the book leave would quickly become another power struggle adding to my anxiety and stress.

Depression is difficult to calibrate for someone who has never experienced it full on. I constantly assessed my symptoms. Gaining those few pounds was surely a good sign. At my next appointment, I pushed Dr. Au for a green light. "I'm okay, aren't I?"

"You're better, but you're not *all* better." She warned I could suffer a relapse if I pushed myself too hard. Disheartened, I began to cry. It never occurred to me that my constant tears were one reason why she thought I hadn't fully recovered.

By late January, with the newspaper putting intense pressure on me to start my book leave, I told Dr. Au that I felt *much* better. Would it be okay to start my book leave? She looked doubtful, especially as I was still weeping at every appointment. I pointed out that I would be working from home during the two-month leave. I suggested this approach might also be rehabilitative: essentially I'd be getting back into writing on my own time and at my own pace, so perhaps when it was time to start again in the newsroom, I'd be up and running.

Dr. Au considered that. Reluctantly, she agreed. When I asked her for a wellness note, she looked surprised. I explained that after all the strife, tension and legal wrangling, I wanted to formally mark the end of my sick leave (even though I had not received any sick benefits or pay since mid-December.)

I felt I needed to draw a line, a wellness line. Unfortunately, I was as ignorant as the next person about depression. The disease is not like that. You aren't sick one day and fine the next. Recovery is complex and not always linear. The wobbly aspect of depression is that, like chronic pain, so much depends on the patient's self-report. I knew I was sick of being sick. When Dr. Au saw how anxious I was, she obliged by writing a brief note. At the same time, she urged me to reconsider taking antidepressants, which in hindsight obviously meant she thought I was still depressed. I left her office clutching the wellness note. I felt neither elation nor a sense of relief. It was all I could do not to cry.

Now that I was officially better, at least on paper, I would actually have to start writing. I did the math: sixty days to pump out ninety thousand words of a decent draft. Could I do it? Much has been written about depression enhancing creativity. I didn't find that to be the case. In fact, that February when I was deeply depressed, I couldn't make much headway on my book at all. I would sit down at my computer each morning, but entire days would go by with little to show for my efforts.

As the days passed, I scolded myself. *C'mon. Snap out of it. Get over it.* I was a journalist, not an *artiste.* Journalists do not suffer from writer's block. We churn it out. When the words slowly began to return, I was euphoric, but wary. One day I managed to write several whole sentences, the next day, a coherent paragraph, then a whole page and then another. When I couldn't sleep, I didn't take a pill. I just got up and wrote more until I crashed with fatigue.

How did I become unblocked after four months? How could I write an entire book, but not newspaper articles? Had my illness been all in my head the whole time? (Of course it had been in my *head*; it was a mental illness, after all.) But was my sudden ability to write again the result of sheer will power? Had I really been able to tell myself to snap out of it? The geographic cure had done some good. So had the music cure. The time away from the office had been healing, too. My family doctor's weekly sessions had been especially therapeutic. Perhaps all these factors had helped me to the point where I could take my first baby writing steps.

But when I think back, I believe there was another more crucial factor: I wasn't writing for the newspaper that I felt had betrayed me. I wasn't creating products for a workplace where problems still festered over whether I had done something wrong in reporting on the Dawson shooting, whether my doctor and I had been lying about my mental health, whether management would ever condemn the racial attacks on me, whether I would ever recoup my withheld sick pay. I was writing this book *for myself.* It was about my search for a Chinese woman I had wronged three decades earlier, and the story itself was redemptive. It was about my own experience, about something that had happened to me in China, long before I had started working at the *Globe.* My book had nothing to do with my employer.

It was the perfect project to bring me back into my old life. As I emerged from the slough of despond and my ability to write improved, I grew increasingly optimistic. Perhaps by the time my two-month book leave ended, I would be in shape to write news and features again.

Even if I had been truly on the mend—and I don't think I was—I could not avoid the stressors that had caused my depression in the first place. I had no buffer from work. Letters (oh, those damned couriered letters!) seemed to arrive with such frequency that I grew afraid to answer the door. In the middle of my book leave, a letter arrived ordering me to undergo a psychiatric assessment. I plunged back into my funk. When I was sick, my workplace didn't believe I was sick. Now that I was better, I had to prove

I had *been* sick. How do you prove that last month you couldn't write?

I was scared. I had never been to a psychiatrist. What if he or she said I had been faking it? "Just tell the psychiatrist what happened," said Dr. Au, writing me a fresh prescription for Ativan. "Cooperate. You have nothing to hide."

I left her office crying anew. I was terrified that the thin stream of words that had returned so slowly and so painfully would dry up again.

PART III

BLUE PRINT

CHAPTER 13

A New Section Called "Life"

Employers who suspect employees of feigning illness can schedule an independent medical exam (I.M.E.). The doctor is not there to treat the patient, but to assess the claim: is it bogus or genuine? As my I.M.E.-date drew near, I became increasingly anxious. I had rejected Dr. Au's suggestion that I see a psychiatrist. Now I was being forced to see one.

I could no longer concentrate on writing my book. Even the simple mechanics of getting to North York General Hospital filled me with anxiety. It was a straightforward route, just ten minutes from my home, but I could not remember how to get there. Like a tourist, I pored over a map. *Turn right out of my driveway. Turn left. Go straight for five traffic lights. Then turn right. Turn left again.*

The night before my assessment, I became stuck in a ruminative cycle. Would the psychiatrist believe me? Try to trip me up? Considering he would be paid several thousand dollars to conduct the exam, would he be beholden to the employer? I lay in bed, rigid, unable to sleep. I didn't take a sedative for fear it would make me incoherent or confused during the exam.

The next morning, I felt very much alone. It was March break, and Sam was on a school exchange, Ben was at his girlfriend's farm and Norman had taken my father to a Caribbean resort. I unlocked the front door of my house and felt the icy air on my face. I'd never really liked driving and, since falling ill, I had avoided it because of the tranquilizers. I gripped the steering wheel of my van so hard the blood drained from my fingers. Everything seemed to unfold in slow motion as I drove along the slippery roads. A late-winter sun glinted off the snowdrifts. The trees looked sharp-edged and surreal.

When I arrived at the hospital, I found all the parking spaces filled, normally a minor irritation. On this morning it seemed an insurmountable crisis. I drove around the parking lot, my anxiety rising as I thought I might be late for my exam. In near hysterics, I finally left my van wedged against a snowbank. With a sense of impending doom, I entered the hulking concrete building. If this sounds over the top, it's because *I* was over the top. In the midst of my depression, the psychiatric exam felt like a kind of judgment day. So much was at stake. If I "failed" the I.M.E., it essentially would mean I had been lying about my illness. My credibility, my reputation and my honor were on the line. At least, that's how it seemed to me.

I took the elevator up to the seventh floor and gave my name to the receptionist. Within a couple of minutes, the psychiatrist appeared. He was fortyish and dressed in a fuzzy sweater and corduroy trousers. His face was round. He did not shake my hand, but his eyes did not seem unkind. He swiped his access pass over a sensor and a heavy glass door clicked open. I had not anticipated a locked ward. When it shut behind us, I felt irrationally afraid. The journalist side said: *of course, they'll let you out, silly.* My depressed side said: *and what if they don't?*

The hall had the blank, bureaucratic atmosphere of an airport security zone. An Asian woman with a baffled expression padded by in slippers and street clothes. I followed the psychiatrist into a windowless conference room. He sat down at one end of a long table and motioned me to take a seat on his left, directly across from a middle-aged woman, whose name I never learned. She smiled encouragingly. She was there to take notes and, I assumed, to be a witness.

"First you have to sign this release," the psychiatrist said, pushing a form across the table. Tears sprang to my eyes. I had paid such a high price for refusing to sign the Manulife authorization form. Was this all an elaborate trick to get me to sign it? At that moment, nothing seemed too far-fetched.

"If you want to think it over, we can postpone this examination," the doctor said evenly.

I shook my head. I had already had one sleepless night. I could not afford to lose any more book-writing time. I quickly read the form and then exhaled. This one was reasonable. It stated that I had agreed to an independent medical assessment and would authorize Medisys Health Group to release the results to Manulife and my doctor. I signed it.

The psychiatrist began by asking dozens of questions.

"How old are you?"

"Fifty-four."

"Where were you born?"

"Montreal."

"Was your birth normal?"

"Yes."

"Do you have learning disabilities?"

"No."

"Do you have a history of psychiatric problems?"

"No."

"Are your parents both alive?"

"No. My mother has passed away."

"What year did your mother die?"

"2003."

"Do you have siblings?"

"Yes. Two brothers and a sister."

"Are you the oldest?"

"I'm second oldest."

"Are you married?"

"Yes."

"How long?"

"Thirty years."

"How many children do you have?"

"Two. Two boys."

"How old are they?"

"Thirteen and sixteen."

"What do you do for a living?"

"I'm a reporter."

"Has anyone in your family ever suffered from mental illness?"

"My mother was depressed, but she talked to her doctor and then she was fine."

"Do you take recreational drugs?"

"No."

"Do you have a problem with alcohol?"

"No."

Then the psychiatrist asked me to tell him what happened. I began by assuring him that I had already recovered and was currently on a book leave. I told him I had three more weeks before I would return to work. Then I began to tell him about Dawson College and the backlash.

To my surprise and confusion, I broke down as soon as I began describing the hate email. Six long months had elapsed since my Dawson story. I was better, wasn't I? I tried to stop crying, but I couldn't. I had prepared a chronology, which kept me on track, even as the tears rolled down my cheeks. Using this outline, I managed to give the doctor the condensed version of what I had told my friends during the long drive to Liz's cottage, adding everything significant that had happened since.

Weirdly, I found I could speak in well-formed sentences, even while weeping copiously. The stenographer kept nodding and smiling encouragingly. After more than an hour of talking and tears, the psychiatrist asked if I needed a break. I shook my head.

"Well, *I* need a break," he said.

I went to the washroom and splashed cold water over my swollen eyes. But back in the conference room, my tears flowed again as I talked about the gag order, the demand that I pay for my old notebooks, the ultimatum to return to the newsroom. After another hour, the doctor looked down at his notepad.

"You keep saying that you are better. But your expression tells me you are not. I think you should consider going back to work only part-time. I don't think you are fully recovered. I think you should consider seeing a psychiatrist."

I began to cry again, out of confusion and despair. When I first fell apart, I didn't believe I was ill and almost no one else did either. Only my family doctor said I was depressed and should not go to work. Then when I realized I *was* sick, my workplace did not believe me. Now, when I thought I had recovered, this psychiatrist was saying I was still sick.

I had been talking and crying for almost three hours. The independent medical exam was over. It was nearly two o'clock when I backed my van out of the snowbank. I drove to a Chinese restaurant and ordered a bowl of noodles, but could hardly swallow a mouthful. Back home, I threw up. I ran a fever. My whole body ached. For the next week, I could barely get out of bed.

In biochemical terms, the danger posed by the psychiatric examination had sent my adrenal cortex into overdrive, flooding my system with cortisol. Instead of running at top speed from the psychiatrist and using up glucose to burn off the cortisol, I had sat rigidly immobile, answering question after question. The fight-or-flight hormone had stalled the work of my digestive system. The excess cortisol had made me vomit to make myself lighter, as the South American black vulture does when fleeing danger. The hormone had also interfered with production of immunoglobulin A (IgA), the antibody that plays a critical role in immunity. With my immune system weakened, I must have caught a bug in the hospital or at the restaurant, hence my fever and aches.

"People who are stressed are more likely to get sick," writes Daniel Levitin. "In contemporary society, increased cortisol levels (and decreased IgA) have been found in experiments conducted during some of the most psychologically stressful situations humans face: students before exams, professional coaches during athletic events, and air traffic controllers during their duty cycle."

When Holli, the clarinetist in my woodwind trio, heard I was sick, she rushed over with two jars of soup, butternut squash and chicken noodle. The soup was all I could manage, and even then, lasted me a week. I was still sick in bed when the phone rang.

"It's David Hayes."

"I can't talk to you," I blurted. "I'm sorry."

Hayes, a freelance writer, had been assigned by *Toronto Life* magazine to write an article about the *Globe* and me. He had already talked to some of my friends and at least one person in management at the newspaper. But I was still under strict instructions not to speak to the media. I was determined to obey until I could get the gag order formally removed from my personnel file. So I couldn't even *tell* Hayes that I wasn't allowed to talk to him because, in the surreal world I now inhabited, I could be accused of talking to him. Norman, who routinely screened my calls, had repeatedly declined an interview on my behalf. But now everyone, including my husband, was still away on March break, and I had unsuspectingly answered the phone.

"Can you talk off the record?" Hayes asked.

"I'm sorry. I can't."

"What about on deep background?"

"I'm sorry, I can't."

I said goodbye, hung up the phone, and went into the bathroom and threw up.

A few days later, fortified by Holli's soups, I was back at my writing desk. With a superhuman effort, I finished the draft of my Beijing book with one day to spare. As my book leave drew to a close, I got the first heartening news in a long time. My "Maid for a Month" series had been nominated for a National Newspaper Award, just the encouragement I needed to return to the newsroom.

Still, I remained anxious. In six months of strife, nothing had been resolved. I still wasn't allowed to respond to the attacks on my family and me. I hadn't received sick pay. And, although three weeks had elapsed since the independent medical exam, I had no idea whether the psychiatrist had supported my claim. Despite repeated requests to the newspaper's human resources department, I had been unable to obtain a copy of my psychiatric assessment.

With a sense of foreboding, I contemplated my imminent return to the newsroom. During the I.M.E., the psychiatrist had suggested I start working only half days. I had rejected that idea, again, because it didn't seem feasible given daily deadlines. I understood the importance of taking a break in the middle of the day, so I carefully lined up a full week of lunch dates with friends. But when I visualized myself walking into the newsroom, I panicked. I confessed to Colleen that I didn't know what to say if anyone asked why I had been away so long.

She drilled me: "How are you?"

I hesitated.

"You say, 'Fine, thanks, and how are you?'"

"Fine, thanks, and how are you?" I parroted.

Colleen said that answer was okay for colleagues, but I should reply differently if a senior manager inquired.

"How are you?" my cousin-in-law prompted.

Again, I was tongue-tied.

"You say, 'I'm doing better.' *Don't elaborate.*"

The morning of my first day back, I made a huge breakfast—bacon, eggs and toast—but couldn't eat. In my absence, I had been transferred into a new section called "Life." I deliberately arrived half an hour early so no one would witness my confusion while I hunted for my desk. I found my spot beside a huge window, a choice location that might signal I wasn't in the doghouse, after all. Switching on my computer, I saw an email from my boss, Cathrin Bradbury, the deputy managing editor of features, who wanted to see me. Nervously, I walked across the empty floor to her office.

"You look great!" she said.

Colleen hadn't prepared me for compliments.

"I've lost a lot of weight," I said awkwardly.

I *did* look great, the old silver lining and all that. I suppose there was little visible indication of the strain I'd been under. Perhaps if I had had cancer, my editor might first have asked how I had been. But what was there to ask? *Still crying every day? Felt like slitting your wrists lately?* The uncomfortable moment passed with the arrival of her assistant. For the next fifteen minutes, the three of us tossed around story ideas. I smiled, I grinned, I cracked jokes. I threw back my head and laughed heartily. I desperately wanted them to believe, I myself wanted to believe, that I was back on track.

I returned to my desk feeling tired and inexplicably blue. Then I smiled. A florist had delivered a tissue-wrapped bowl of roses and sweet peas. "Welcome back!" the card said. "Love, a loyal reader." The flowers were from the nicest hockey mom on the Finland/Sweden trip, the only one in whom I had confided. Her kind gesture cheered me up immensely and gave me the courage to sort through my backlog of correspondence.

Suddenly I noticed a fresh email from human resources:

The results of the Impartial [sic] Medical Examination has [sic] been received and reviewed. The results are that the absence for the period December 12, 2006 to January 26, 2007, the start of her book leave, is supported.

I exhaled and split into two. Their psychiatrist had upheld my claim. I was not a liar after all. I would finally receive my sick pay and the long dispute would end. The journalist side noted the irony: I was relieved, thrilled even, to learn I had been genuinely ill.

My workplace seemed a drearier, sadder place. For the first time, I was conscious of the soul-destroying hues: dried-blood and hospital-green walls, gray polyester cubicles. I began to notice that colleagues rarely said hello or made eye contact as they passed in the hall. At lunch (when I was dashing out to see friends) I saw my fellow reporters and editors carrying Styrofoam clamshells of cafeteria food back to their desks to eat in silence. I watched as they emailed coworkers who were sitting a few feet away. I had previously ascribed this behavior to deadline pressures. It now struck me as dehumanizing.

The environment hadn't changed, of course. Depression merely offered a new lens through which to view the world. My illness had given me insight into the dark side, into the triggers for depression all around me. This is the gift—and the curse—of depression. You begin to see your surroundings as they really are. You are no longer blind. It's like that snippet of Chinese fortune-cookie wisdom: optimists believe we live in the best of worlds and pessimists fear this is true.

Depressives see their glasses as always half empty, which some would argue is a more accurate and realistic view of the world around them, especially if they toil in a toxic workplace. In "Mourning and Melancholia", Freud suggested that depressives have "a keener eye for the truth." Andrew Solomon describes a study in which depressed people who played a video game for half an hour knew precisely how many monsters they had slaughtered whereas those who weren't depressed guessed four to six more than they had actually killed.

Kyla Dunn, a freelance journalist and former biotech researcher, calls this phenomenon "depressive realism." Depression is not the near-death experience described by so many, she suggests, but a rebirth in which the new psyche has removed self-delusion. Compared with so-called healthy individuals, depressives are more realistic in their worldview. "One cognitive symptom of depression might be the loss of optimistic, self-enhancing biases that normally protect healthy people against assaults to their self-esteem. In many instances, depressives may simply be judging ... the world more accurately than non-depressed people, and finding it not a pretty place."

Take workplace friendships, for instance. Work had been the defining structure of my life. My obsession with work had fooled me into misconstruing professional relationships as personal friendships. I thought I had many friends in the newsroom. But as months passed, it dawned on me that if I wasn't at work, I no longer existed—for these friends. From my isolated vantage point, it seemed as though the camaraderie of the workplace had vanished at the first whiff of trouble. Or I thought perhaps the stigma of depression was affecting co-workers, too, and they preferred to stay safely away. When I was ill, only a handful of colleagues got in touch. At least, that's how I remember it. Many later told me they had no idea what was going on because I hadn't said anything.

People who have experienced depression often become more empathetic to the outside world (even while remaining angry and narcissistic with family). I must have radiated empathy once I was back in the newsroom. Colleagues began telling me their own stories. My friend, Val Ross, organized drinks after work with two other *Globe* reporters. Over glasses of merlot at Le Sélect Bistro, they assured me I wasn't alone. The three, all women, revealed that they, too, had been sick from work-related stress. Val told me she had been taking antidepressants for years. When I said I was frightened of meds and hadn't taken them, she smiled. "It's the only way I can stand working here."

I had always admired Val. She was a brilliant journalist who had covered the literary beat and later worked as an editor on the Op-Ed page. It shocked me that she had been depressed. She certainly didn't look it. But that was the problem, wasn't it? A depressed person can look like her, a beautiful, elegant, successful woman with a captivating smile and a mischievous sense of humor.

My colleagues' depression was largely hidden from view. But some workplaces are so lethal they end up in the headlines. At France Télécom, the world's third-largest telecommunications company, forty-three employees killed themselves between January 2008 and February 2009 after the second-in-command, dubbed "Cost-killer," engineered the layoffs of 22,000 employees. Several left suicide notes explicitly blaming the workplace. "Cost-killer" resigned and the entire management team was replaced. An interim report commissioned by Télécom warned that the new management team had to address the suicide crisis and "encourage radical change."

For surviving employees, a toxic workplace can exact a serious toll. Researchers at the University of Manitoba found that the emotional cost of workplace bullying now surpasses that of sexual harassment. Victims of bullying are becoming ill from anxiety, depression and post-traumatic stress disorder.

At least one in three American workers has experienced bullying on the job, according to a survey by the research firm, IBOPE Zogby International. The harassment can be as trivial as a smirk. It can include belittling comments or an amused shake of the head every time the victim says something at a meeting. It often involves repeated failure to return calls or answer email, "forgetting" to include someone in an important meeting, assigning a project doomed to fail or stripping someone of critical duties and then accusing them of not doing the job.

A brilliantly conceived research project is following the health and career of more than ten thousand British civil servants, a perfect cohort because everyone has an identifiable rank, yet access to the same quality of medical care. Since 1967, the Whitehall Studies have found that the lower the rank, the higher the incidence of various illnesses, including high blood pressure, heart attacks and depression—just like the baboons Sapolsky studied.

The insurance industry is feeling the hit. Manulife Financial Group—yes, the same Manulife company intervening in my sick leave—calls mental-health claims the fastest-growing category of disability costs in Canada, according to *Benefits Canada*, a trade publication. Manulife, a global insurer that operates in the United States as John Hancock Financial, blames the soaring cost of antidepressants and anti-anxiety drugs. It says that lost productivity for mental illness in Canada alone costs more than $8 billion a year.

At the beginning of my second week back, I began receiving fresh hate email. Someone shot forty-nine people at Virginia Polytechnic Institute and State University, the worst school shooting in U.S. history. The perpetrator fit the pattern: he was a young, depressed male who, at the end of his rampage, committed suicide.

"Quick! Send Jan Wong to Blacksburg..." J. Lépine emailed me.

Someone named André emailed, "Notice to all: Jan Wong isn't a journalist at the *Globe and Mail* but only *une pauvre cloche anti-francophone*" ("a pathetic anti-francophone dumbbell").

I hadn't written a word about Virginia Tech. Why was I getting more hate email? Then I discovered someone had been impersonating me in a chat room on a *La Presse* website. "My" comments had provoked a fresh onslaught of vitriol. Running to the washroom, I locked myself in a stall and began to cry.

At my weekly appointment with Dr. Au, I told her I had changed my mind. I wanted to see a psychiatrist, after all. Could she refer me? I assumed it would take months to see one and I wanted to get on a waiting list in case things kept deteriorating at work.

"Are you sure?" she asked.

Her question surprised me. Hadn't *she* wanted me to see one?

"If you ever want to work in management," she said, "you won't be able to. The human-resources department will eventually find out you've seen a psychiatrist."

CHAPTER 14

Shrink-Fit

The *Toronto Life* feature hit the newsstands my second week back at work. It appeared under the headline, "Notes on a Scandal." Nervously, I scanned the story. I was now so crazed I had to read it through three times before I could understand it. Hayes had called me a "diva" and the editor-in-chief a "dope." He called my *pure laine* charge "explosive" and said my piece on Dawson had "ignited a firestorm." The *Globe* had not supported me against the backlash. Its "crime," he added, was to "run for cover and let its star reporter take the fall."

A few days later, I was summoned to a meeting in the executive boardroom. The vice-president of human resources, flanked by the deputy editor, read from typed notes. She said I had disobeyed orders not to talk to media. Specifically, she said I had talked to Hayes.

But I hadn't and I said so. I concentrated on not crying.

"Then who did David Hayes talk to?" the human resources vice-president asked.

I said I didn't know. I suggested that she ask Hayes. At that point the deputy editor jumped in. She asked if I had shown my friends any of the letters the company had sent to me. I nodded. "All my friends know what has happened to me," I said. I had been distraught when my sick pay was halted at Christmas, I explained, and had confided in those closest to me.

The deputy editor now ordered me not to talk to my friends about "internal company matters." She wanted the names of each friend I had talked to. I declined to name names. It felt surreal. Was it even legal for an employer to bar someone from talking to her friends ... about herself? I felt claustrophobic, panicky and cornered. I held my tears until I after I got back to my cubicle.

Twenty-four hours later, I returned to the same boardroom to celebrate the launch of the new "Life" section. The polished mahogany table, where I had so recently been interrogated, now held bottles of Champagne and a huge bowl of strawberries. About twenty staff stood with their backs against the wall, eating tasteless strawberries as big as golf balls. No one was sure what to do with the little green tops, so people clenched them in their fists.

It was the classic office party, where everyone remains alert and watchful while trying to appear witty and relaxed. I stood alone, feeling chilled.

I was still processing what had happened to me the previous day when the publisher came over to exchange pleasantries. He smiled at me. I smiled back. It was like a bad dream. First, they drive you nuts; then they make you eat out-of-season fruit.

Much later, I would see a verbatim transcript of that boardroom meeting, a strong indication that it had been secretly recorded. At the time, I sensed that the vice-president of human resources had been reading from a script provided by a lawyer and so the next day I hired my own lawyer. Sort of. My lawyer could do no more than advise me from the sidelines because, under Canadian law, union members are not allowed to have independent counsel when dealing with their employers. As time passed, even my relationship with the union and the union's lawyer became increasingly fraught. And then my lawyer had to start advising me on how to deal with my union, too.

Not surprisingly, given the fresh hate emails, the *Toronto Life* article and the boardroom meeting, I seemed to be falling apart again. To my immense relief, the psychiatrist to whom I was referred by Dr. Au phoned to say he could see me immediately. I had waited only one week. In contrast, the average wait time for a psychiatrist is seventeen weeks, even though the Canadian Psychiatric Association recommends a delay of no more than four weeks for patients with major depression.

I went to my first appointment that Monday after work. The discreet sign outside his office, on the twenty-ninth floor of a gleaming bank tower, indicated only that he was a medical doctor. He shared the tiny waiting room with another doctor, who had an equally vague exterior sign. Once I was inside, it became clear that the second doctor specialized in cosmetic injections and dermal-filler treatments to soften wrinkles. The journalist in me thought: *how convenient—one-stop shopping for stressed-out people.* In addition to talking about your worries, you could Botox your worry lines, too.

I was relieved to find the waiting room deserted, without even a receptionist. Like many psychiatrists, my new doctor managed his appointments himself. He later told me that his patients didn't like dealing with a third party. (There it was again: the centuries-old stigma that the patients themselves had unconsciously internalized.)

I sat down in a soft, caramel leather armchair and averted my gaze from the copy of the day's *Globe and Mail* on the side table. Instead I stared at the pale-green walls. A classical radio station played Haydn softly through small, high-quality loudspeakers. I heard a distant ping and the sound of a heavy door closing. Suddenly a door swung open and the doctor was standing there. He motioned me into a small anteroom and through another door into his office. The setup reminded me of a high-security mantrap, of the kind used by banks in Rome to control entry. The doctor's was designed with discretion in mind. The double sets of doors seemed intended to thwart eavesdropping and inadvertent glimpses of the patients on the other side.

His huge, irregularly shaped office had spectacular floor-to-ceiling views of Lake Ontario and reminded me of a living room in a two-million-dollar penthouse. It felt empty, despite a large, green leather couch, two leather swivel chairs, two desks, some plants, a wall of filing cabinets and a bookshelf. Sixteen framed diplomas and certificates hung on the wall (although it would take me two years of appointments before I regained my journalistic abilities enough to notice and count them).

The doctor gestured toward the couch. I hesitated. Was I supposed to lie on it, as in a *New Yorker* cartoon? I sat down instead. He sat opposite in one of the swivel chairs. The gap between us seemed unnaturally wide. Was this to preserve a professional distance? Or was it to give the doctor a fighting chance in case I lunged at him with a hatchet?

Bruce Menchions appeared to be in his forties or early fifties. He had a bushy brown beard, streaked white down the center. He wore khaki pants, a pressed cotton shirt and walking shoes. Somehow he managed to look simultaneously friendly, unthreatening and detached all at the same time. I liked him on sight. In fact, I liked him so much that many months later I committed a psychiatric faux pas. I was feeling hungry before an appointment and bought a box of Belgian chocolates. When I offered him one from the opened box, he recoiled. It dawned on me that one of the first rules they're probably taught at shrink school is never to accept candy from a patient. (Poison, hidden razor blades—you get the drift.)

Psychotherapy is only effective if you like your psychiatrist *and* your psychiatrist likes you. By the time I learned this, I had been seeing Dr. Menchions for more than a year. I asked him what happens when the therapist dislikes the patient.

"Some Jewish doctors don't like it if a patient is anti-Semitic," he told me.

Had he ever disliked a patient?

He gave me a psychiatric-survey type reply. "I think I've actively disliked fifteen to twenty out of a thousand. Some of them called me 'fat.' Like if they're talking about exercise, they might say, 'Oh, you wouldn't understand because you're fat.'"

"Well, I *am* fat. But I would try my very best to be professional. Only once, I had to ask a patient to find another doctor because it wasn't working." (I wouldn't call Dr. Menchions *thin*, but he is not fat. I felt bad on his behalf when he revealed this to me.)

I've since learned that several of my friends tried out a psychiatrist or two, disliked them and gave up on any treatment at all. Andrew Solomon sampled eleven therapists in six weeks and writes that he finds it incredible that people will drive an extra twenty minutes to use a favorite dry cleaner, but aren't choosy when it came to a psychiatrist. "Remember, you are at the very least placing your mind in the hands of this person."

That Solomon sampled eleven therapists seems mind-boggling, but then I don't even have a dry cleaner. I was lucky I clicked with Dr. Menchions. When I once slipped up and called him a "shrink," he didn't take offence. "People have called me worse things to my face," he said, shrugging off my apology.

At my first session, I did not know the protocol. I did not even know what psychiatrists did or how they could help. Did I talk, or did he talk? I looked at Dr. Menchions, waiting for him to take charge.

"How are you?" he said, looking at me through wire-rimmed glasses, investing each word with warmth and meaning.

To my embarrassment, I burst into huge sobs. There were boxes of tissues on each side of the couch. It didn't occur to me until much later that both psychiatrists and HR professionals always keep a box of tissue handy for clients. I grabbed a tissue, and then another. Even as I dabbed my eyes, I split into two: distraught patient and cool observer. Did the after-hours cleaner ever wonder why the wastebasket in this particular office was always filled with damp, crumpled tissues?

Just as I had done with the psychiatrist at the independent medical exam, I launched into the short version. I said I had already recovered from depression and was determined to resume my normal life. I told him about the *Toronto Life* article and how I'd been blamed. I explained that I had been neglecting my children and my husband, and that I sometimes took my anger out on them. I cried throughout. The doctor listened intently, gently interrupting when I had gotten only part way through my story. The allotted fifty minutes had elapsed.

"We need to set up another appointment," he said. "I think I should see you again in a few days."

To my surprise, Dr. Menchions showed me out through a different door. Then I understood. A separate entry and exit prevented psychiatric patients from bumping into one another. The exit was set up in the same mantrap style as the entrance. The first door led to an antechamber no bigger than a closet, which led to a second door—this one unmarked—opening onto the outer hall. All those doors, all that wasted space, another nod to that age-old furtiveness about mental illness. As I stepped through the second door and turned to say goodbye, I suddenly remembered that I wanted to reassure my doctor about something.

"By the way," I said, smiling wanly, "I'm not planning to kill myself."

CHAPTER 15

Relapse

This is how Dr. Menchions filled out the psychiatric form at my first appointment:

IDENTIFYING DATA: National reporter – Globe & Mail
PRESENTING ISSUE(S) depressive symptoms 2° work sit'n
HISTORY OF PRESENT ISSUE(S) – onset over past few months:
- Insomnia
- Dysphoria
- Focus/concentration ($\downarrow$)
- Anhedonia
- Loss of appetite – weight loss
- Withdrawal from family
PSYCHIATRIC HISTORY – 0
HISTORY OF PHYSICAL HEALTH – well
PERSONAL AND FAMILY HISTORY:
- stable marriage
- unremarkable developmental milestones.
- Religion – sophisticated view of life
- History of street drug, prescription drug, or alcohol abuse: 0
- Outstanding legal or significant financial difficulties – 0 other than work
- Other identified unusual experiences, exposures or pressures –
  Dawson College opinion – backlash in media, mentioned in
  Commons, was misunderstood, misinterpreted
MENTAL STATUS EXAMINATION
- Appearance – younger than age; appropr. dress
- Behavior – good eye contact; dysphoria/weeping
- Cognition: subj.report – $\downarrow$- focus/conc.
- Speech: articulate
- Affect: v. sad (MDE) – can "put on a front" professionally
- Thought: 0 thought disorder, but fears may have some cognitive distortion
- Suicidal ideation: passive only, fleeting, 0 plans (not in my opinion at
  elevated risk)

FORMAL DIAGNOSIS:
AXIS I: <u>MDE</u>
AXIS II: – (normally very assertive and inquiring)
AXIS III: –
AXIS IV: work
AXIS V: GAF: 50 now, apparently 85-90 normally

Most people never see their psychiatric file. I obtained mine for my legal battle over my unpaid sick benefits. Even though the clinical notes were about me, I felt pained, slightly voyeuristic and creeped-out when I read them more than a year later. It was nice to hear that I had a stable marriage, a sophisticated view of life, and, yes! that I looked younger than my age. But it jolted me to see, in black and white, Dr. Menchions's unequivocal diagnosis of major depression. A trained and experienced psychiatrist had expressed no ambivalence at all. The same was true of my family doctor and the psychiatrist at the independent medical exam. When I read through Dr. Menchions's notes, I had to look up "dysphoria," which is a fancy word for sadness. I wasn't familiar with "anhedonia" either; it describes an inability to experience pleasure. "M.D.E.," which Dr. Menchions had underlined, stood for "Major Depressive Episode."

The formal diagnosis for depression consists of five axes, as specified in *DSM-IV*. These five axes provide a standardized system for communicating a mental-health diagnosis to hospitals, clinics and insurance companies. Axis I covers major psychiatric disorders, including depression, anxiety, bipolar disorder, ADHD, phobias and schizophrenia. Axis II covers personality disorders such as paranoia, narcissism, obsessive-compulsive disorder and what is still called "mental retardation." Axis III covers medical conditions and physical disorders, such as brain injuries. Axis IV looks at psychosocial and environmental factors contributing to the disorder.

Axis V concerns global assessment of functioning (GAF), a number that particularly interests insurance companies because it quantifies an individual's psychological, social and occupational functioning. In short, it assesses the ability to work. Calibrated on a scale of 1 to 100, a GAF score of zero is vegetative. A GAF score of 50 or less signifies severe depression. There is no "passing grade," but insurers often rule that a score of 60 or 70 means the patient is well enough to get off disability.

At my first session, Dr. Menchions assessed me at 50 and estimated I needed a GAF score of 90 to perform my duties as a journalist. In other words, I remained severely depressed even after I had returned to work. At the time, he didn't tell me that his diagnosis was M.D.E. Perhaps he could see that I would resist. At my second appointment, however, he suggested antidepressants. I refused, just as I had with Dr. Au. It would take nine more appointments before I would fully accept his diagnosis and two more months *after* that before I would finally agree to try medication.

Now, two years later, having written the chapter about the trip to Scandinavia, and having remembered the perceived coldness of the other hockey parents and how I clung to Sam, I see that it should have been obvious to me that I was in the grip of a serious mood disorder. But the terrible cruelty of the affliction is that the person who is depressed can hardly see anything clearly. Denial is part of the trap of depression, part of its insidious nature, blinding the sufferer to the illness spreading from within. For eight months, from September to April, I had told myself I was merely sad. I didn't know that the criterion set out in *DSM IV* is two *weeks* of sustained symptoms, including depressed mood, diminished interest in normal daily activities, loss of appetite, inability to sleep, fatigue, feelings of worthlessness and diminished ability to concentrate.

When Dr. Au had suggested antidepressants, I had burst into tears. That should have been a clue all by itself that I was clinically depressed. Instead, I sought counter-evidence in stereotypes. I wasn't wandering around the shopping mall in pajamas. My hair wasn't matted. I bathed. I smiled at appropriate moments. How could I be depressed?

"Can 'put on a front' professionally," Dr. Menchions had noted. At work, I *was* putting on a good front. I had been role-playing the old me, going to meetings, coming up with story ideas and trying so hard to get back to normal, to my successful and happy life as a reporter.

A few weeks after I returned to work, the *Globe* finally issued a check for the six weeks of sick pay the company had stopped from mid-December to the start of my book leave. I didn't expect an apology, and there was none. I hoped, however, this would mark the end of the dispute. Instead, management continued to courier more letters to my home. Smiling, the deputy editor personally dropped one off at my desk. It summarized the meeting over the *Toronto Life* article, a meeting I now dubbed "my boardroom interrogation." To my distress, this letter went into my personnel file, too.

I had been back at work for six weeks and was feeling deeply depressed. Despite repeated requests, I still hadn't been able to see the psychiatrist's report from my I.M.E. The deputy editor had just vetoed a story I'd written about Conrad Black, the former newspaper baron. The four-thousand-word feature had been assigned to me, and it was a scoop. It was the kind of controversial story the paper loved. No one would tell me why it was killed. I sat despondently at my desk. My writer's block returned.

As the date of the National Newspaper Awards dinner neared, I grew increasingly anxious about the prospect of spending a whole evening fraternizing with senior management. But I was determined to attend, if only to prove to myself that my career was not on life support. The *Globe* was flying every nominee and spouse to the gala in Winnipeg, so I casually mentioned it to my husband. Normally, he'd rather have a root canal than attend a black-tie dinner. Would he go with me?

"Sure," Norman replied.

I thought I had misheard. This particular black-tie event meant flying three thousand kilometers to listen to some self-absorbed journalists natter about their work. (He already had that last bit at home.) Just as I hadn't understood why my son, Ben, had uncharacteristically bought me tickets to the symphony, it didn't occur to me why my husband so readily agreed to go with me to the awards dinner. Much later, when I asked why, he said, "I thought you needed someone to take care of you."

With my accrued sick pay suddenly swelling my bank account, a new symptom suddenly, ah, materialized. I began shopping. Before my illness, I had enjoyed the occasional outing to the mall. Now shopping became a compulsion. I could not go into a store without buying something, anything. I wasn't even safe in the supermarket. If I encountered someone offering samples of ready-made pasta dinners, which I never ate, I bought several packages anyway. I also bought books, pots and pans, socks, underwear and lipstick, even though I don't wear lipstick.

One day I bought a ridiculously expensive, skimpy, black silk cocktail dress. Let me put this in context: I have never before owned a cocktail dress, skimpy or otherwise. And here's the proof—is this too much information?—I didn't even know how to shave my armpits.

Subconsciously, I probably viewed the dress as armor for my upcoming evening with management. That hazard, however, paled in comparison with the terror of my first-ever waxing appointment. Colleen had booked an appointment for me at a salon called Planet Nails. A white-coated technician ushered me into a back room and pointed to a high bed that looked alarmingly like an operating table. I clambered on. At her instruction, I dutifully raised my arms above my head so she could inspect my armpits. Then she stared down at my face.

"Would you like your eyebrows and lips waxed, too? We have a special."

I didn't have a mustache, but as an Asian, I am genetically programmed to lunge at specials. Or perhaps it was one more symptom of being depressed; I just wanted to spend money all the time. If the technician had offered to wax my tongue, I probably would have agreed.

"Okay," I said.

"Close your eyes."

Neurobiologists who study primates have found that social grooming reduces tension and stress. My waxing session therefore had great therapeutic potential. *Rip!* Had she just skinned my forehead? Before I could protest, I felt a searing pain as she painted my upper lip with molten wax. She laid a bandage over my mouth and ripped again. Next, she splashed scalding coffee on my underarms, or at least, that's how it felt. *Rip!* The technician gave me a mirror to inspect the damage. My armpits were bald. My eyebrows looked unnaturally neat. And my upper lip looked red and angry. I was ready for my big night out.

Norman and I took a morning flight to Winnipeg, which happened to be the same flight my editor-in-chief was on. That made me so anxious that by the time I got to Winnipeg in mid-afternoon, I just wanted to crawl into bed. Unfortunately, I had more primate grooming scheduled. My sister had urged me to get my hair styled for the dinner and I had forty-five minutes before my appointment in the hotel's salon. I told Norman I needed to take a nap. Would he wake me at the right time? He explained he wanted to go out exploring because he had never before set foot in Winnipeg.

"Why don't you use your alarm clock?" he said, quite reasonably.

"What if the clock doesn't work?"

"Then call the front desk and ask for a wake-up call."

"What if they forget?" I countered, verging on hysteria.

"All right," he said, with only a trace of grumpiness. "I'll wake you up."

It's amazing that he didn't divorce me. If I could have divorced myself, I would have. At home, Norman had been picking up the slack. When I couldn't get out of bed, he made breakfast and roused our teens for school. He did the laundry. He made me lunch, even though I only picked at food. He screened every phone call and took messages that I never returned. He agreed instantly to anything I suggested, whether it was a walk around the neighborhood, a movie or an expedition to the grocery store, where he would push the cart behind me and act as my assistant. *Pick six pears, good ones, no bruises. We need bleach.*

Exactly forty-five minutes later, Norman returned from his walk and woke me up. If only he'd had ten more minutes, he grumbled, he could have made it to the gravesite of Louis Riel. I barely paid attention. Everything was about me.

Downstairs at the hair salon, a young man with blue hair and many tattoos teased my hair into a ludicrous bouffant. Upstairs, I slipped on my new cocktail dress. I practiced walking around the room in my new high-heeled Ralph Lauren mules, purchased during my Arizona trip with Dad. In the bathroom, I applied bright-red lipstick I'd bought for the occasion. I admired my bald armpits. I practiced smiling at the mirror. I positively sparkled. I looked successful, enviably thin and glamorous (except for the 1960s bouffant hair). That was the outside. Inside, I was quaking. I was close to tears. I felt no confidence at all.

With Norman sticking close by, I went downstairs to the ballroom and entered the crush of journalists. There was a red rose corsage for each nominee. I badly wanted to wear mine so everyone would know I wasn't a failure, but my skimpy dress left nowhere suitable to pin it. I stuck it inside my evening bag where it wilted.

A short, middle-aged man I didn't recognize reached out his hand. "I'm André Pratte," he said. I shook it and smiled. A nanosecond later I realized he was the editorial writer at *La Presse* who had written the commentary that appeared later in the *Globe* attacking me ("*Pure laine* is pure nonsense.") Pratte had since been promoted to editor-in-chief. My smile was still frozen on my face when he announced, "I have a great idea for a series. There's going to be a federal election. We want to send you with one of our reporters across Canada. You'll go together to different cities and write stories about each place. We'll translate your stories and publish them side by side with ours. Your paper can do the same."

It was a provocative concept and normally I might have gone for it. But I couldn't take another Internet stoning, not at the moment. "You'd better talk to my editors," I said, turning away.

Thankfully the *Globe*'s editor-in-chief stayed far away, but the tuxedo-clad publisher spied me from across the room. Suddenly Phillip Crawley was at my side, giving me an enthusiastic hug and air kiss. I smiled as if on autopilot, inwardly recoiling. This was the CEO of the company that had silenced me, frozen my sick pay and refused to run my stories. I wondered: *how does he condone my treatment?*

I had never paid much attention to the newspaper's corporate hierarchy. After spending months ruminating at home, it occurred to me that the vice-president of human resources reported directly to the publisher and was unlikely to do anything without his approval. I noted that she had filled a vacancy created when the publisher married the newspaper's *previous* vice-president of human resources. The entwined relationships belatedly struck me as ominous. My piddling troubles, however, were clearly the last thing on the publisher's mind. He was ebullient because the *Globe* had garnered thirteen nominations, more than any other newspaper.

After cocktails, we sat down to huge slabs of beef and salmon. The dinner—and the awards—seemed to take hours. My category, long features, was nearly the last to be announced. The maid series was up against a *Toronto Star* story by Mitch Potter on Canadian troops in Afghanistan and a feature on poverty by a team from *La Presse*. I'm so petty I prayed that *La Presse* wouldn't win, and they didn't. Mitch did. Afterward, I went up to congratulate him.

"I really needed to win," I said, only half kidding.

"I've never won one," he said, giving me a hug. "You already won one."

I didn't think anyone remembered. I sighed. It seemed a lifetime ago.

I wasn't the only *Globe* loser. Despite thirteen nominations, the newspaper took home only four awards. Later, in the newspaper's hospitality suite, the publisher made a speech about how the judges had lacked judgment. Everyone duly chuckled. Norman couldn't take any more and retreated to our room. I should have called it a night, too. Instead, just as I had refused to budge at the luggage carousel, I willed myself to stay at the post-dinner reception. I sat on a couch on the far side of the room, slipped off the designer mules and flexed my sore toes. A moment later, the publisher sat down beside me. Why did it feel like he was always homing in on me? For the next half hour, he talked to me about everything except Dawson. He was charming. I nodded and smiled and nodded some more.

That night, I was so agitated I couldn't sleep. The next morning, I woke up exhausted. Norman was still muttering about missing Louis Riel's grave. When you've been married for thirty years and your spouse complains long enough, you eventually hear him. I proposed we stop off at the site on our way to the airport.

"What if it's not on the way?"

"Then we'll leave twenty minutes earlier," I said.

St. Boniface Cathedral was indeed on the way. Riel, who was hanged in 1885 for leading a rebellion, had the place of honor in the cemetery. As every Canadian schoolchild knows, Riel was Métis, the mixed-race offspring of a French father and an aboriginal mother. In my depressed, narcissistic state, I viewed everything through the prism of my troubles: Riel, hero of French Canada, was not *pure laine.*

Depression affects cognition. When you're in the midst of a major depressive episode, your judgment is compromised. I should have known better than to expose myself to so much stress. The previous evening had been too great an effort and I was about to suffer the consequences. My system was flooding with cortisol. I was on the brink of a breakdown.

On Air Canada Flight 258 to Toronto, Norman and I were unable to get seats together. He sat further back, giving me the better spot, an aisle seat in the first row in economy. I was watching *The Painted Veil*, starring Naomi Watts and Edward Norton, when the personal screen in front of me suddenly went black. The crew had switched off the video system.

The woman beside me hadn't finished her movie, either. "I can't believe they turned it off so early. We're not going to land for another half hour," she groused.

"I'll ask why," I said, leaping into my investigative-journalist, fight-for-the-underdog mode. That was the old me, always championing causes, even trivial ones. Actually, I'd been thinking of writing about the precipitous decline in airline service, ever since a flight-attendant friend told me she had picked up two new skills at her annual August refresher course: defusing bombs and tying up terrorists. Shutting down the video system mid-movie looked like a promising place to start. I pushed the attendant-call button.

The purser, a tall, blond and deeply tanned man, loomed over my seat. I asked why the movie had been stopped so early. "We shut it down because we have to collect the headsets," he said, clearly irritated at being summoned for such a pointless question.

Alas, the occupational hazards of being a reporter include (a) knowing useless information and (b) hating when people lie to you. I told the purser that couldn't be the reason because Air Canada now lets passengers keep the headsets.

"It's a security regulation," he snapped.

We were on a collision course, an overworked flight attendant and a pesky, depressed reporter. I pressed further. How could shutting off the movies possibly involve security?

"What are you, twelve?"

I expected the woman beside me to speak up, but she stayed silent and averted her eyes. In my depressed state, I perceived that as another betrayal. My pulse racing, hardly able to breathe, I noticed the purser had a French-Canadian accent. Ever since Dawson, that accent sent me into a panic, sparking a flashback of Internet stonings, racist attacks and death threats. Trembling, I barreled ahead.

"Why don't you warn passengers at the beginning of the flight that they won't be able finish the movie?"

"Madam, honestly," he snorted. He turned to other passengers for support. "Who is right, me or her?" he asked.

"You are," shouted one passenger, who also had a French-Canadian accent. My heart began thumping wildly. I tried to hold back my tears. I could no longer speak.

"See? At least *some* customers are nice," said the purser. Apropos of nothing, he said, "I saw how many carry-on bags you had. You had four bags."

I didn't have four bags, but I couldn't manage to say anything more than, "What's your name?" Stepping back into my reporter role, I began scribbling notes on the margin of the in-flight magazine.

"No names," said the purser, enraged.

To my relief, the seatbelt sign clicked on. He left to start preparing the cabin for landing. As the plane banked, I saw him strap himself into a jump seat in business class. Then, ignoring the startled looks of other passengers, he began blowing kisses down the aisle at me, big, fat, sarcastic kisses.

I could not believe this was happening. The only explanation I can muster is my theory that depressed people radiate a kick-me aura. When I later discussed this with Dr. Menchions, he agreed. "Some people do. And some people have the radar to hear it," he said. "Bullies, especially. In any kind of predatory activity, the predator tries to select the victim. They read the signals. They watch body language. Who shies away? Who won't look you in the eye? They don't always get it right, but predators often sense which kid is weak."

On this Air Canada flight, the purser wasn't finished with me. He blew one more sneering kiss and then shouted down the aisle, "You can't leave when we land."

"Why not?" I shouted back, trying to keep my voice strong. I braced myself for arrest. Anything seemed possible.

"Because hospitality wants your name. I'm going to take your name."

With my last bit of psychic energy, I shouted my name and spelled it for him. That finally shut him up. Sometimes flight attendants recognized me, or at least my name, after I'd written a story about smuggling box cutters onto four Air Canada flights in the aftermath of 9/11. For whatever reason, the purser abruptly stopped talking and ignored me as I deplaned.

Once I was in the terminal and the purser could no longer see me, I couldn't stop crying. Was I really unraveling over a rude flight attendant? Or was I having a time-delayed meltdown from the night before? One of my colleagues, a business reporter, had been seated too far back to overhear the altercation. Now he caught up with me as I hurried through the terminal. Mystified, he tried his best to comfort me. Norman, too, caught up with us and was equally perplexed by my tears. I sobbed all the way home. Between gulps and gasps, I tried to tell my husband what happened.

"Don't take it so hard," the taxi driver said kindly, turning around in his seat after he had pulled into our driveway. "Lots of my customers hate Air Canada."

CHAPTER 16

Running in the Family

Once home, I collapsed. That night, I had a nightmare about another glittering, black-tie dinner with the editor-in-chief and the publisher. It ended with the three of us riding a cable car off a cliff.

Robert Sapolsky's research shows that baboons with sustained high levels of cortisol have trouble distinguishing between situations that are life threatening and those that are mildly irritating. Right under a tree heavy with fruit, these over-anxious baboons will fight to death over a single banana. On the Air Canada flight, I had disintegrated over the in-flight movie—in primate terms, a banana.

By chance I had already booked Monday as a day off. On Tuesday, I phoned in sick because I couldn't stop crying and went to see Dr. Au for more sleeping pills.

"The I.M.E. report arrived," she said, passing me a manila envelope.

I had waited nine weeks for this. Now, my heart pounding, I quickly scanned the eight-page report. On the last page, this paragraph leaped out:

Ms. Wong appears motivated to return to work at this time. I suggest in the interest of facilitating a productive and sustainable work return that this be done with the utmost consideration to her emotional wellbeing and while being mindful of the fact that her condition is in partial remission at this time.

That "utmost consideration" had not happened. Instead the company had interrogated me in the boardroom and put the follow-up letter in my file. It had not published my Conrad Black feature, and would not tell me why.

Partial remission. So that's why everything had seemed so dreary at the office, why I had found it so difficult to cope. I had gone to the Winnipeg awards thinking it would mark my return to normalcy. Instead I had come back a soggy mess. If only it hadn't taken so many weeks to see this report, I might have been more cautious about returning to work. I might not have gone to Winnipeg.

The I.M.E. report concluded: "If she begins to experience a relapse of her depressive symptoms, I would suggest a referral to a psychiatrist and a reconsideration of the use of an antidepressant."

I felt both relieved and shattered. Reading the report was a key moment in my depression. A psychiatrist, paid by my employer to assess me, had ruled I remained depressed. So had my family doctor and my own psychiatrist. After months of resistance, I finally accepted the diagnosis, stigma be damned.

At my next appointment with Dr. Menchions, I showed him the I.M.E. report. He wasn't surprised by its contents. He listened as I told him what had happened in Winnipeg and how I had disintegrated over a stupid in-flight movie.

"GAF remains at 50," he wrote in his notes.

He again urged me to start a regimen of antidepressants. This time, I nodded tearfully. He wrote out a prescription for a popular new drug called Cipralex, also known as Lexapro (generic equivalent, escitalopram). And then he wrote his first sick note for me. I would not be going back to work.

Like my family doctor, Dr. Menchions informed my employer I needed two weeks off. Unlike Dr. Au, he described me as "completely disabled from work."

Completely disabled. Those two words startled and frightened me. Until then, I thought "completely disabled" meant someone in a wheelchair. On my way home that evening, I filled the prescription at the first pharmacy I passed. Deep down, I still hoped I would not have to take any meds. I believed that the unequivocal I.M.E. report would convince my employer that I was genuinely sick. The company would of course act compassionately and responsibly. Then the strife would end and I could get well.

I submitted my psychiatrist's note to human resources. Within hours, I received by courier the same blurry Manulife form I had refused to sign the last time. The union's grievance over the form was still grinding its way through the arbitration process. It would be another month before the union would win, forcing the corporation to adopt a new form. In the meantime, human resources gave me forty-eight hours to sign the old form. Otherwise my sick pay would be stopped. Again.

I let the deadline pass.

A courier delivered a second letter, with another ultimatum. This time human resources gave me twenty-four hours to sign. I let the second deadline pass. The next week, my sick pay and all benefits were stopped, all over again.

Dr. Menchions was perplexed. He told me he had never seen an employer, react like this to one of his sick notes. I fell deeper into the abyss. With a feeling of hopelessness, I swallowed my first antidepressant, a white, oval 10-milligram dose of Cipralex.

That day was Sam's fourteenth birthday. Did I bake him a cake? Did he have a party? Did I buy him a present? I can't remember. The tentacles of depression ensnare a sufferer's loved ones, too, leaving them bewildered and often angry. I became aware of how absent I had been. But at least, I told myself, I never stopped feeding my family. I would make pots of spaghetti, duck *confit,* standing ribs of beef, even if I hardly ate anything myself.

Two years later, when I sit Sam down to ask what this time was like for him, he pours a glass of milk and sighs. He tells me I'm wrong when I say I prepared lavish meals for the family. "You didn't cook *forever.* I had to cook meals for so long. Every day. Pasta, stir-fries. Ben would do the dishes." In fact, Sam had stepped in and baked a chocolate cake for one of Ben's birthdays because I couldn't get myself organized. "It took hours." He sighed again.

How had I fabricated an image of myself cozily tending the hearth even as the rest of my life collapsed? Was my false memory self-protective? When Sam tells me this, the real memories return in a rush. I can see him at the stove and Ben leaning over the sink. I feel shocked and guilty. Not only did I neglect my children, I can't even recall that I did. I do remember the constant rage. In normal times I have a short fuse. When I was sick, I veered out of control. I either foamed at the mouth or was emotionally absent. I was completely immersed—drowning, really—in my own problems and I took it out on those I loved.

"Depression will bend you out of normal restraints," Dr. Menchions later explained to me. "Your behavior becomes more extreme because more extreme things are happening to you."

I ask Sam what else he remembers. "At the beginning, I didn't know you were depressed," he says slowly. "I just thought you didn't want to go to work, that you were being unreasonable."

I digest this, trying to see it from my son's point of view. When he was little and said *he* was feeling sick, I'd check his temperature. If he didn't have a fever, I'd invariably pack him off to school. Of course, I *didn't* have a fever and my symptoms were much harder to pinpoint, so his lack of faith doesn't sting. After all, at the beginning of my depression *I* didn't believe I was sick either, so how could I expect Sam to have seen the signs or even know what they were? I didn't see them with my own mother. I now bitterly regret that I never talked about it with her, not when she first mentioned it when I was a teenager, not in the last year of her life when she was wasting away.

At one time or another, virtually every family will be impacted by depression. But the taboo has left these same families ignorant and vulnerable. For a pervasive disease, depression remains diabolically hidden. Until I succumbed myself, I had no idea that one in five or six people will get it. Untreated—and as we've seen, half won't get any treatment—depression can lead to abuse and familial breakdown. In the worst cases, men who are depressed beat their wives. Occasionally, they kill their entire families (or storm into a school and shoot everyone in sight).

Marriage protects against depression, but once it occurs it puts a tremendous strain on all relationships. One in four marriages will break up if one partner is depressed. Virginia Woolf captured this estrangement in her novel *Mrs. Dalloway*. Septimus, a shell-shocked survivor of World War I, is told by his unhappy wife, Rezia, that she is lonely and wants to have a baby: "Far away he heard her sobbing; he heard it accurately, he noticed it distinctly; he compared it to a piston thumping. But he felt nothing. His wife was crying, and he felt nothing; only each time she sobbed in this profound, this silent, this hopeless way, he descended another step into the pit."

Studies of depressed mothers show that their babies have distinctive brain-wave patterns. Most infants lock eyes with anyone who coos at them. Babies of depressed mothers turn away and exhibit a lack of interest in their environment. They display unhappy facial expressions and have slow motor movements that persist beyond the two-week minimum specified in *DSM IV*, the psychiatric manual.

Older children of chronically depressed mothers often do poorly academically. The same year I became sick, Sam was placed on academic probation. When his guidance counselor called me into the school to give me the bad news, I cried. (Okay, his math mark was *really* bad.) I blamed everything on myself. Depressives, imprisoned in narcissism, are typically consumed with guilt because, of course, everything is always about them.

"I don't think that was your fault," Sam said later. "I felt bad about that because you were blaming yourself. It was just me. You probably *weren't* taking care of me. Frankly, when I'm thirteen it doesn't matter if you tuck me in."

Was Sam right? Had he, at thirteen, been fully responsible for his poor academic standing? Or had my illness undermined his performance? Arnold Sameroff, a developmental psychologist at the University of Michigan, concludes that children adapt because they understand when their parents are incapacitated.

For his part, Ben responded to near-total maternal neglect by working extremely hard. In the two years that I was sick, he went from Mr. Mediocre to the Headmaster's List. He aced his final exams, won the English Prize and was accepted at every university to which he applied. Ben's success doesn't exonerate me. Not only did I fail to help my kids when I was sick, I often took my anger out on them.

"You were freaking out and screaming a lot. Over more stupid stuff," agrees Sam. He remembers being jolted awake one night by my shrieks. "You were trying to throw Ben's laptop out the window. I took it and hid it from you," he said. "Then I talked to you for an hour. I had to be, like, the 'peace guy' for that one. You went back into Ben's room to say you were sorry, but he was asleep."

Memories surface from my own childhood. My mother, who was prone to terrible rages, too, once snapped at me to be quiet. I can't remember what I was nattering on about, only that it was incredibly important to me at the time. Had my mother been in the midst of a depression, too, unable to focus on anyone but herself? I see myself, perhaps ten years old, seething with indignation. I'm sitting in my bedroom with the gauzy white curtains and the delicate, violet floral wallpaper my mother had let me choose myself. I'm hunched over my large white desk. With my best fountain pen, I write a solemn oath in Waterman blue ink on a small sheet of white paper. It's a secret vow, so I tuck it under my bright blue desk blotter. I write: "I promise that when I'm a mother I will always listen to my kids."

I broke that promise. Instead, I made my children listen to *me*. I ask Sam if it was terrible for him. He laughs. "I'd rather be the peacemaker than the one getting his laptop thrown out the window." He adds that I often screamed at him, too. In Sam's case, our fights were over my demands that he accompany me to a movie, any movie.

"I didn't want to go. Ben would say, like, 'She has depression, so you have to go.'" Sam would reluctantly acquiesce. He reminds me of the embarrassing time I glommed onto him and his friends at the movies. "You tried to sit next to us. But there were not enough seats. So you sat across the aisle. It was kind of weird."

Apparently, his friends never teased him about his strange mother. Perhaps thirteen year olds think all parents are bizarre. Or maybe they sensed somethin was off and pitied Sam. At first he did not confide in his friends. "It was an illness. They didn't need to know."

But with me leaning so heavily on him, my son eventually had to lean on his friends. "I just brought it up one day," he says. "'So, um, my mom has depression.' I told them what happened, about the article you wrote and the death threat. They were like, 'Oh.' They felt bad."

When Sam tells me that, I feel a surge of hope. Were his teenage friends too young to have assimilated the cultural stigma? Or was it easier for them to accept my depression because by then *I* had accepted the diagnosis and was open about it? I know that when one of Sam's classmates was later hospitalized for depression, the boy chose to confide in him. He knew Sam would understand.

Even though I was emotionally absent during my depression, it was a relief to know my son had a support group that provided what I couldn't— comfort and understanding. His classmates didn't avoid me the way it felt that my colleagues did. In fact, they were more empathic than most adults. The boys—and the occasional girl—would drop by for juice and cookies, burgers, leftover pasta and Chinese chive dumplings. They came over almost every day to play basketball or road hockey in our driveway. The noisy exuberance of galumphing teenagers helped rouse me from my stupor. It made me happy to watch them eat when I couldn't.

Apparently the ever-present swarm of companions was also a protective shield for Sam. "You'd put on your fake nice face and you wouldn't scream at me." But whenever he was alone with me, he felt a need to escape. "That's why I was always going to friends' houses and having sleepovers all the time. In grade seven, I would stay at school for an hour and a half after classes because I didn't want to come home."

I taste regret and loss. It never occurred to me that Sam couldn't bear being at home. What was it like having a crazy person for a mother?

"It was just annoying. I felt I had to be good and helpful. I had to be pleasant when I came home. So I'd just go in my room and pretend to do homework," Sam says, finishing his glass of milk. "One of the things I noticed when you had depression was that you wouldn't just get mad. You had mood swings. You could be happy and have fun, but then someone spills a piece of pasta on the table, you would just flip the table. Then ... *flamethrower in my face.*"

For the record, we don't own a flamethrower. And although my memory is faulty, I'm pretty sure I didn't actually flip the table. Or did I? I'm about to ask Sam when he gives me that *are-you-done?* look. He gets up, ready to escape. My throat constricts with a spasm of love. I want to give him a bear hug. Instead I stand there, willing myself to keep my arms at my side. As I recover, I'm finally able to respect his need for space and independence. But at sixteen, he still needs direction. I nod at his empty glass.

"Put that in the dishwasher," I say.

When I was sick I was so difficult to talk to, so nervous and edgy and volatile. Ben did not tell me about the night he was assaulted on the street. Instead, he shared it only with Norman (who also decided it was best not to say anything to me). "You would have overreacted," said Ben, two years later, when he finally mentioned the incident. He had been biking across an intersection in an upscale residential neighborhood one evening when a drunken teenager, a passerby, suddenly sucker-punched him in the stomach. Shocked, Ben dismounted. The kid then slugged him in the chest and finished with a head butt. Although Ben hadn't been seriously injured, he was understandably upset at the random, unprovoked stranger assault. I felt bad about that, but even worse that I hadn't been there for my son. It underlined for me how absent I had been. I was home, but I might as well have been on Mars.

What is the difference between the family's recollection of these dark days and my own? They remember the whole picture while I remember only fragments. Oddly, I mostly recall the positive bits, like the time Ben took me to the symphony. I also remember that, as my resident IT expert, my son offered to block unwanted email from the *Globe* during my illness. After he saw how certain missives threw me into a tailspin, he told me, "I can program it to block anything from work." He could bounce back email unread, delete them right away or send them to a file to read when I felt better, whatever I wished. Ben was so reassuring and calm, a younger version of his father. At the time, I was conscious only of his helping me. I had nothing left to understand the emotional underpinnings of his efforts. Ben was trying to be a man, stretching to protect his helpless mother. But instead of responding with love, I screamed at him.

Throughout this time, Norman was a steadying influence on the boys and on me. I had grown up in a family of four siblings who were always fighting over the window seats in the family Chevrolet or the last dish of chocolate pudding at supper. Norman, an only child, was not used to internecine strife. But when I was sick, he would listen patiently to my ruminative rants, over and over and over again, without ever once telling me to shut up. When the boys were really upset with me, they would seek solace from him.

"Well," he would tell them with a deep sigh. And then he would say nothing for a long time. He'd look quizzically at the boys through his glasses. Then he'd sigh again. "There's nothing you can do about it. She's not well. Try to be understanding and accommodating, as much as you can." That would calm them somewhat. His sighs told them he commiserated with them. His words told them they were doing the right thing.

On occasion, I would be so unreasonable, so crazy, that I would push my long-suffering husband right over the edge. Then he would stomp out of the room (without slamming the door as I would have done). An hour later, he would be back again, calm, steady and hovering in the background. He never retaliated.

I phoned Gigi to ask what she recalled about the fights with my kids. She remembered the laptop incident vividly. "You called me, screaming." Apparently I had needed help with a computer problem and Ben had been on the phone with his girlfriend. I had waited and fumed and waited some more. And then, after he finally got off the phone, I exploded.

"He wanted you to say, 'please,' and you wouldn't, so he wouldn't fix your computer," my sister recalled.

That night, Gigi said, Ben couldn't handle it any longer. "He couldn't stop crying. I asked him if he wanted to get away from you. I told him he could come to Montreal any time. That's when I decided I'd better come to Toronto to help you with the arbitrations."

I didn't remember that either. I only knew that at a certain point, my sister was by my side. She was unconditionally there for me. She phoned nightly. She organized my legal files. She came to Toronto at every critical juncture. For two years she had refused to speak to me, had cut me dead, had refused to take my calls. Now she stood shoulder to shoulder with me, helping me through the biggest crisis of my life. My tattered relationship with her had not only mended, it had grown stronger than before. Gigi would be my therapist, financial advisor, legal strategist, marriage counselor, travel companion and life support. In short, she became the best sister in the world.

It was not without cost. My sister had plenty of her own pressures, including helping her son settle into university and overseeing her daughter's applications to medical school. And Dad, with whom she lived, was slowly deteriorating. He began having trouble with stairs and sometimes lost his balance. Gigi developed a blister in one eye from all the stress. Each time she had to leave Dad alone in Montreal to help me in Toronto, she worried about him, and he worried about both of us. My illness had damaged my whole family. Yet I could not have survived without them.

Not surprisingly, depression is thought to be worse in modern Western society because of divorce, rootlessness and the demise of the extended family. More than any other people in the world, Americans move from job to job, city to city and even from one place of worship to another. They have the highest rate of divorce and romantic breakup on earth. By age thirty-five, one in every ten American women will have lived with three or more husbands or partners, a higher proportion than women in Europe, Canada, Japan, Australia and New Zealand.

In Asia, by contrast, the family structure remains strong. Married sons in China commonly live with their parents. After giving birth, a new mother is pampered for the first thirty days, barred from doing any cooking or housework while family members arrive with nourishing foods to ensure her milk is flowing. The result: strikingly different rates of postpartum depression—just 4 percent in China, compared with about 10 percent in the West.

Incidentally, a limited but growing body of literature indicates there may well be male postpartum depression, too. Fathers, of course, are not affected by hormonal fluctuations related to childbirth, but they are subject to the same psychosocial stressors that accompany new parenthood. The very few studies to date show wildly different estimates—between 1.2 and 25.5 percent. Nevertheless, the incidence of depression in new fathers appears to be higher than in the general adult male population, according to James F. Paulson, a psychologist at Eastern Virginia Medical School in Norfolk.

Paradoxically, depressives vent their anger on those closest to them, even as their sadness sensitizes them to the needs of others. While I was horrid to my family, I was kindness incarnate to strangers. I'm not normally all that considerate, but I began holding doors open for everyone. I responded to any appeal—heart and stroke, cancer, epilepsy, multiple sclerosis, the Daily Bread Food Bank, McGill University, World Vision, UNICEF, Human Rights Watch. In the subway, I threw coins into the violin cases of buskers. If I saw a pregnant woman or anyone at all who looked tired, I would give up my seat on the subway. I would haul baby strollers up and down flights of stairs. I would walk confused tourists all the way to the correct platform.

In a department store, I once escorted a blind woman from the basement to the second floor so she could buy a sweater. Along the way, I named the merchandise we were passing.

"Now we're going through the perfume section."

"Yes," she replied drily. "I know."

Helping strangers made me briefly happy. If you didn't know what I was like at home, you would have thought I was an angel.

CHAPTER 17

Cipralex, Celexa, Effexor, Wellbutrin

My return to work had been a false dawn. The realization that I'd had a relapse devastated me. My life began to revolve around my weekly psychiatric appointments. "Work issues are unquestionably contributing to prolonging symptoms," Dr. Menchions wrote in his clinical notes. Technically it wasn't a relapse, he said, but a continuation of the original depressive episode.

Either way, the statistics were grim. Those who suffer from a severe depression have a 50 percent chance of having another. And if the first episode is severe and prolonged enough, it can actually alter the brain's physical structure. "It's becoming clear that in the hippocampus, the part of the brain most susceptible to stress hormones, you see atrophy in people with post-traumatic stress disorder and major depression," writes Robert Sapolsky.

Scientists have repeatedly found significant brain pathology when conducting scans of patients with depression, schizophrenia or manic-depression. "It is possible that repeated psychosis or depression may exacerbate the already fragile chemistry of a vulnerable brain," says Kay Redfield Jamison. I don't know what was happening to my brain's physical structure, but I know I felt unremitting stress. With my sick pay stopped for the second time, the union offered to make me available for another I.M.E. And now that I was no longer afraid of psychiatrists, I was more than willing to go. But the second time around, the company refused.

The union then filed a grievance over the second withholding of my sick pay. It filed more grievances over the new disciplinary letters in my file and the same old Manulife authorization form (which I was still being pressured to sign). Mediations and arbitrations were scheduled. Lawyers were consulted. The company sent more letters to me by, yes, courier, which particularly gnawed at me. Perhaps to the company it was merely paperwork, but to me it seemed spitefully symbolic: it was so quick to halt my sick pay, and yet so ready to waste ten bucks every time it sent me a letter.

Once chronic stress throws your biochemistry out of whack, anything and everything becomes a stressor, even a stupid couriered letter. The more episodes of depression you suffer from, the worse they get and the more frequently they occur. Think of the first episode as being like a dislocated shoulder. If you are not careful and you dislocate it several times more within a short period, your shoulder will eventually slip out of place without a tug. When depression becomes chronic, it no longer requires an external kindling event. It's like the dislocated shoulder that spontaneously pops out of its socket.

Without medication, there is as much as an 80 percent chance of a relapse within a year. But choosing the right antidepressant is a random, messy business. Dr. Menchions warned that the drug could take a month or more before I felt any improvement in mood. Half the time the first one won't work. Unfortunately, you still have to wait from four to six suspenseful weeks to be sure it's not working and then gradually step down the dosage, under your doctor's supervision, while introducing the next drug, which also has a 50 percent chance of being ineffective.

Nevertheless, insurance companies would rather pay for drugs than for talk therapy because drugs are cheaper. As doctors, patients and insurers all search for a chemical solution to every problem, antidepressants have become the best-selling drugs in America, even more common than headache pills. Cymbalta, Paxil, Lexapro, Zoloft, Effexor, Cipralex and Prozac hold the top spots; Tylenol, in contrast, is way down the list, in twenty-second place. Today America spends $10 billion a year on antidepressants, the most of any country in the world. Sales also have surged in countries as diverse as India and New Zealand. At the same time, people without medical insurance, including many in the United States and in developing countries, have little or no access to medication. In 2009, a University of Pennsylvania study polled 250 Philadelphia homeowners on the brink of foreclosure and found that more than one-third suffered from major clinical depression. But fully half of them were too poor to pay for medication.

Psychotropic drug therapies were introduced in the 1950s. The boom in sales began in the 1970s, with the introduction of Valium. In the late 1980s, Prozac went on sale, the first blockbuster SSRI (selective serotonin reuptake inhibitor). Today, SSRIs are the most widely prescribed psychotropic drugs. In Canada, from 1999 to 2003, the number of SSRI prescriptions rose by 80 percent to 15.7 million. By 2008, there were 22.6 million prescriptions, according to IMS Health, a private company that tracks drug sales.

As noted earlier, serotonin, a neurotransmitter, plays a mysterious role in depression. Nerve cells release serotonin to facilitate the transmission of signals. Once the signal has been transmitted, the nerve cells typically reabsorb or "reuptake" whatever serotonin is left. SSRIs work by blocking this reuptake, thereby keeping more serotonin sloshing around in the brain.

Having more serotonin afloat in the brain seems to improve mood, even though there is no scientific evidence that a "deficiency" of serotonin causes depression in the first place. (An oft-cited analogy is that aspirin relieves headaches, but a low level of aspirin doesn't *cause* headaches.)

Effexor, another popular antidepressant, was introduced in the 1990s. It works on serotonin and norepinephrine (noradrenalin), both implicated in depression. Meanwhile a third type of antidepressant, called MAO-A inhibitors, is regaining popularity. Originally favored in the 1970s and 1980s, it inhibits a protein found in the brain called monoamine oxidase A that appears to be a factor in recurrent depressive episodes. MAO-A inhibitors have unfortunate side effects, including sexual dysfunction, but they do increase the levels of norepinephrine and serotonin afloat in the brain.

Intensive marketing by pharmaceutical companies has sparked the boom in antidepressant use. Increased usage could also be a sign that people are now addressing their psychiatric problems. Critics, however, say drugs only make it easier for people to dodge the underlying problem. Others oppose medication on the grounds that unhappiness is a natural and inevitable part of life. I disagree with the critics. Unhappiness is certainly part of life, but unhappiness is not the same as clinical depression. For the severely depressed, the medications may boost you to the point where you have the insight and energy to solve your problems and make healthy life changes.

No one yet knows the long-term health effects of taking antidepressants. The longest study of Effexor lasted only two years, even though many people stay on it for a decade or for life. Nor is all the research that has been conducted readily available. In 2008 the *New England Journal of Medicine* scrutinized seventy-four clinical trials involving twelve antidepressants. It found that 97 percent of positive studies were published, but only 12 percent of negative studies. According to the same article, drug manufacturers failed to publish the results of one-third of all antidepressant trials submitted to the U.S. Food and Drug Administration from 1987 to 2004. When these unpublished trials are included in the calculation, the drugs' performance turns out to be lackluster. More than half, or 57 percent, failed to show a statistically significant difference between the antidepressant and an inert placebo.

On instructions from my psychiatrist, I started with a daily 10-milligram pill of Cipralex, a relatively new (and expensive) antidepressant in the SSRI family. It was touted as having fewer side effects. I deliberately avoided checking it on the Internet. I figured that reading about potential side effects was a pretty good guarantee I'd develop them. After a short time my eyes became so dry I had to use drops. My mouth felt parched no matter how much water I drank, a concern because lack of saliva causes gingivitis and tooth decay. I noticed other problems, too. At my Monday-night band rehearsals, I could no longer keep the beat. My fingers became unresponsive. I couldn't remember the key signature. At home, I became clumsier than usual, knocking over coffee mugs and brushing cutlery onto the kitchen floor. While talking or eating, I would accidentally chomp down on my cheeks until the inside of my mouth was swollen and raw.

Nine weeks of Cipralex, my first psychotropic drug, failed to lift my mood. So Dr. Menchions reduced the dosage while starting me on 20-milligrams daily of Celexa, an older (and cheaper) SSRI. Unfortunately, the side effects were the same as before, with the addition of hot flashes that left me breathless, and with even worse memory lapses.

On Celexa, I felt like someone had stuffed cotton balls into my brain. Even before my Air Canada meltdown, I had had trouble remembering appointments. Now it was as though I'd lost my mind. Correction: I had misplaced my mind and couldn't remember exactly where. I forgot to lock my front door. I lost my checkbook. I even forgot that my woodwind trio was coming over to rehearse and went out to meet a friend instead. One Wednesday night I went to a flute choir practice as usual, remembering that it had been canceled only after I got there. I forgot Sam had a math tutor coming to the house. I forgot that Ben had a fiddling lesson. And this was all in one week.

I would find mysterious events listed in my datebook, but have no memory of arranging them. "You'd call and say, 'Did we book lunch?'" said my friend, Paul, who works at a bank. I kept missing appointments. Terrified, I began using a fluorescent-orange marker to highlight every important item in my datebook. I would review my schedule the night before and check it again the next morning. Unfortunately, my brain could not retain any information for more than a few minutes. I missed an important ophthalmologist appointment. I also forgot to show up for two sessions with Dr. Menchions, despite anticipating each one like a drug addict awaiting her next fix.

At one session, I was trying to describe a friend's brother but couldn't find the word. "He's, um, what do you call it? An alcohol addict."

"Alcoholic," my doctor reminded me.

After the first month on Celexa, I was still in the black hole. Dr. Menchions doubled the dose to 40 milligrams and warned, "If your memory worsens, go back to one pill."

It was in fact difficult to say whether Celexa was improving my mood because my situation at work was getting worse. Maybe the SSRI was merely keeping me from the screaming meemies. I stayed on Celexa for four months and still felt very low. My doctor decided to try another drug, Effexor, also known as venlafaxine. It was the same antidepressant that Dr. Au had suggested I take in the first place.

I took Effexor for six months. As part of the SNRI class of antidepressants, Effexor works by inhibiting reuptake of both serotonin and norepinephrine. To my dismay, a new side effect emerged. Or rather, didn't. All-Bran, my usual cure, was useless. As Norman so tactfully put it, I was full of shit. When I developed painful hemorrhoids, Dr. Menchions suggested Preparation H, which did little except make me feel geriatric. He then recommended drinking milk of magnesia, a thick, chalky cream that tastes exactly like it sounds. When that didn't work, he proposed Metamucil, a Tang-like drink, which, when inexpertly mixed, left disgusting gelatinous lumps at the bottom of the glass. I remained severely constipated, plus now I gagged on the drink that was meant to be a cure. (Those lumps really got to me.) Prowling the drugstore shelves, I finally found the solution: Bowel Buddy Bran Wafers. (Slogan: "The permanent solution to flushing.") The straw-like slabs—the word "cookies" was a euphemism—cost sixteen dollars a package, but I became a loyal consumer.

Aside from my delight at finding Bowel Buddy, Effexor failed to improve my mood. Ten months and three meds later, my psychiatrist weaned me off it and switched me to Wellbutrin, also known as bupropion. Under the brand name Zyban, it is often prescribed to help people stop smoking. Categorized as an "atypical" antidepressant, Wellbutrin works by inhibiting the reuptake of two neurotransmitters, norepinephrine (noradrenalin) and dopamine. I stayed on Wellbutrin for five months, taking two 100-milligram pills a day. It gave me heart palpitations, but to my relief, my severe constipation ended and I could at last say goodbye to my Bowel Buddy.

In all, with overlapping drug regimens, I spent fifteen months on meds. Did they help me? The unequivocal answer is: I'm not sure. The first three drugs, Cipralex, Celexa and Effexor, did nothing (although in hindsight perhaps they kept me from becoming bedridden). It's possible that the last one, Wellbutrin, had some salutary effect. Then again, my recovery might have been entirely the result of months of psychiatric counseling. Or perhaps my depression had run its course. With or without treatment, depressive episodes typically last eight months. Mine lasted more than two years.

I write this as if the sequence and schedule of medication was clear.

It wasn't. If you had asked me at the time what medication I was taking, I couldn't have told you. I had round, Smurf-blue pills; tiny white ovals; large, flesh-colored, blister-packed gel capsules filled with white powder; and teensy, dull-white lozenges. To write this account, I relied on pharmaceutical receipts and empty pill containers and my medical file. In twenty-three months, I had twenty-nine prescriptions for antidepressants, anti-anxiety medications and sleeping pills.

I would wander into whichever drug store I happened to be passing and hand over a fresh prescription. The pharmacist would glance pityingly at me and hand over a sheaf of pamphlets covering such topics as "Sexual Dysfunction and Depression."

"Have you taken these before?"

Nod.

"You know you can't have alcohol with them?"

Another nod.

Sometimes I took one pill a day, sometimes two. Sometimes I'd be decreasing the dose of an old antidepressant while starting a new one. I had so many pill bottles they would tumble out when I opened my medicine cabinet. With my memory on the fritz, I had trouble remembering whether I had taken the day's pills or not. I began keeping my meds in a clear plastic pillbox, the elongated kind the elderly use, with snap-up lids and separate compartments for each day of the week. Mine was in French, English and Braille, in case I also went blind.

With cortisol flooding my brain again, it was either fight or flight. Were I the male-school-shooter type, I might have chosen fight. But I chose flight, hoping I could pull that off by pretending to be a tourist in my own city. I took a walking tour of my neighborhood. I visited the site of Canada's first parliament (now a carwash). I went downtown and, guidebook in hand, inspected the granite carvings of busy bees and thrifty squirrels on the cornice of an old bank building.

When the stay-at-home vacation didn't help, six or seven friends jumped in with invitations to their cottages. Then an Australian journalist in Paris emailed me. We didn't know each other, but she had heard about my troubles through a mutual friend. As a gesture of solidarity, she invited me to stay in her flat in Montmartre while she was away visiting her parents in Australia.

Three weeks in Paris. My heart lightened. But the moment I booked the flight, I began to feel guilty. If I was too sick to work, shouldn't I be too sick for Paris? The stigma of depression is so insidious that even while ensnared in its black jaws, I remained prejudiced against the cure that had helped me before.

Dr. Menchions encouraged me to go. "It will be therapeutic."

I felt so lucky to have found a psychiatrist like him. I noticed that on his business card, he had listed an MBA in addition to his medical degree. One day I asked why he hadn't gone into the corporate world.

"I didn't agree with what I saw," he said.

My psychiatrist treated me with medication and therapy, a combination which researchers say works better and faster than either on its own. At first I didn't know exactly what the fifty-minute sessions did for me. All Dr. Menchions seemed to do was sit and listen to me talk. (Ben was amazed that you could get paid for that, which seemed way easier than his after-school job of walking our neighbor's dog, Mickey.)

"I provide constancy, something that you can count on," Dr. Menchions said, more than a year later. "You can trust it. The goal is to get you to be as comfortable as possible so you can share things."

It *was* infinitely therapeutic to know I could talk and someone would listen, someone who wouldn't be driven away because I kept repeating myself ad nauseam. I counted the days and hours until my next visit. The relief provided by talk therapy would last only a few days, until I received another letter from work. William Styron waited until he was suicidal to see a psychiatrist. He wrote that the doctor "at least offers consolation if not much hope, and becomes the receptacle for an outpouring of woes during fifty minutes…" Neither his experience nor mine means that the sessions were pointless. Pain relievers wear off, too, but no one ever suggests that's a reason not to take Tylenol 3.

Even though I interviewed people for a living, I couldn't imagine being on the receiving end of a depressed person's monologue, week after week, month after month, year after year. After I'd been seeing Dr. Menchions for four months, I had a nightmare. In it he blurted that I was the most boring patient he'd ever had. Chagrined, I asked why.

"Because all you ever do," he answered with a snort, "is talk about yourself."

Occasionally, during a late-afternoon or early evening appointment, my psychiatrist's eyelids would droop. Once, I was tactless enough to remark on this. Dr. Menchions sat bolt upright, apologized instantly and looked so mortified that I never mentioned it again. Instead, I became like an after-dinner speaker trying to keep my audience of one awake. I strained to be witty and animated. I juiced up my anecdotes, sharpened my commentary. I had never cared much if my bosses liked me, but for some inexpressible reason I really cared that my psychiatrist did.

Apparently, most patients try to impress their therapists. They see it, rather pathetically, as their last chance for approval. "I sit up straight and I don't cry," Solomon wrote of his attempts to impress various psychiatrists. "I represent myself with ironies and interject gallows humor in a peculiar effort to charm the ones who treat me, people who do not in fact wish to be charmed."

Psychiatrists don't want to be your friend, hence the twelve-foot seating gap. Dr. Menchions would start every session by warmly asking, "How are you?" That was the signal for me to launch into my monologue. Once, it occurred to me to politely reply, "How are you?" My doctor looked surprised, and then said he was fine. I became curious to know whether other patients ever asked him the same question. He thought for a moment, and then gave me another psychiatric-survey type reply. "Maybe seven in a thousand."

At first, I didn't understand why any expertise was required to merely sit there like a sounding board. I later understood that my psychiatrist was not passively listening. He would interject a sentence or two at strategic moments, when he judged the time was right. At one session, for instance, as I recounted the latest blows inflicted on me, I wondered aloud whether I was being paranoid.

"You're not paranoid," he said firmly. "Paranoia is a pathology and yours is based on experience." If my workplace had been supportive, he added, I would have already recovered. It made me feel somewhat better to hear that. At least I was beginning to understand why I was sick, which was part of the journey to getting better.

The kind of psychotherapy Dr. Menchions provided is called cognitive behavioral therapy, or CBT. At just the right moment, he would give me a mental nudge, the way a rocket is fired to alter the trajectory of a missile so it avoids smashing into Earth. For instance, when I blamed myself for Sam being on academic probation, my doctor told me that guilt is a major symptom of depression. That simple fact improved my mood. At least I now knew *why* I felt guilty.

"I wait around to say the thing that matters. It's all timing, art, finesse. But it isn't trickery," he said. "There are no hard statistics on psychotherapy except that we know that a patient must have some kind of belief in the therapist's ability."

Talk therapy—the practice of revealing risky personal thoughts—emerged from Freudian psychoanalysis in which the patient reclines on a couch (that couch!) and uncovers early trauma by talking for five or six hours a week for years on end. Dr. Menchions told me he underwent psychoanalysis himself as part of his psychiatric training. I couldn't imagine talking about myself that much—although I'm sure Norman would say I already do.

Psychoanalysis itself derived from a ritual of the Catholic Church. "The Catholic confessional is a brilliant mechanism to expose what troubles you, what you're most ashamed of. And you can come back the following week and confess to exactly the same thing. The priest is not censorious, but embracing," said Lionel Tiger, anthropologist and co-author of *God's Brain*. Inside the confessional booth, sinners unburden themselves in confidence. Not that they necessarily obtain quality advice. In his novel *Madame Bovary*, Gustave Flaubert sends his adulterous, severely depressed heroine to her priest, who can only murmur platitudes. Emma Bovary eventually swallows arsenic and dies an agonizing death.

Edwardian England served up similar platitudes to depressives. In *Mrs. Dalloway*, Virginia Woolf describes how Septimus has become suicidal after witnessing a friend and fellow soldier blown to bits on the battlefield. Dr. Holmes, his blustery English physician, tells Septimus he's just fine. "For he had forty years' experience behind him; and Septimus could take Dr. Holmes's word for it—there was nothing whatever the matter with him."

Unlike poor Septimus, I knew that I was clinically depressed. Two of my own doctors and the psychiatrist who conducted the I.M.E. had said so. Unfortunately, their opinions didn't count. Manulife's did. And as my intervention specialist told me over the phone, early in our oddly intimate, oddly distant relationship, "I've been doing disability assessment for thirty-two years. You're not sick." Only much later did I realize that she had echoed the fictional Dr. Holmes.

CHAPTER 18

The Upside of Being Down

The paradox of depression lies in its prevalence. Shouldn't Darwinian natural selection have bred it out long ago? Depression is so punishing, yet so common. Given that one in every five or six people suffers from depression, why are we as a species still are so prone to this debilitating illness?

But what if depression is *not* a weakness or a defect? What if it's Nature's way of protecting us so that we can regain our health to live another day? Could depression be a defensive mechanism against chronic stress? After all, we are the descendants of those who, on hearing the snap of a twig in the forest, learned to withdraw from danger.

Evolutionary psychologists have suggested that getting depressed could be a *cri de coeur*, a way of making others aware of our distress. My inability to perform the daily tasks of a reporter was an involuntary response to intolerable stress. My psyche had gone on strike, so to speak, to protest working conditions that included hate email and death threats.

Sadness, Darwin wrote, "leads an animal to pursue that course of action which is most beneficial." Perhaps overwhelming sadness is a shield. When you're depressed, you withdraw from everything, especially the stressful situation that made you sick in the first place. Perhaps the paralysis, the retreat from the world, shelters depressives from the immediate threat and gives them breathing room to regroup. Darwin himself speculated on the evolutionary purpose of his own misery. "Pain or suffering of any kind, if long continued, causes depression and lessens the power of action, yet it is well adapted to make a creature guard itself against any great or sudden evil." Depression could be a serendipitous time-out, a breather or a forced respite for those of us too busy to stop and take a realistic inventory of our lives. Depression gives us a chance for introspection. Problem solving follows, along with the development of a new perspective and, upon recovery, reintegration into society. Isn't that the story of every mythical hero's adventures?

So ... what if depression is beneficial in evolutionary terms? What if it's actually *good* for humanity? The British psychiatrist Paul Keedwell has suggested that depression does have a positive side. "The truth is that short-term pain can lead to longer-term gain," he writes. In his book *How Sadness Survived*, Keedwell cites a study of depression in the Netherlands that found that most people coped better with adversity *after* experiencing depression. The survey, conducted in three waves, in 1996, 1997 and 1999, surveyed ordinary Dutch people aged eighteen to sixty-four. Their lives improved significantly following recovery from depression, compared to before the onset of the illness, in virtually every area including vitality, psychological health, social and leisure activities, occupational performance and general health. The biggest surprise was that the severity of depression and the availability of treatment were not significant predictors of functional decline. Among the minority who got worse after a depressive episode, the most important factors were social isolation that pre-dated the depression and co-existing conditions, such as drug abuse or physical illness. In short, after suffering from a depression, most people coped better with life's trials. Consider it the upside of being down: we do not suffer in vain. Now, if only we could overcome the stigma and talk openly about depression, we might gain a more acute appreciation of the human condition and learn how to weather adversity.

Although depression is an emotional illness, people crave physical evidence. Certainly, they expect you to *look* depressed. "Psychomotor retardation"—moving and talking slowly—is one of the few visible symptoms. But it is by no means a universal symptom. Indeed, it's often impossible to tell from outward appearances whether someone is depressed or not. Recall that after Wade Belak committed suicide, his NHL coach said the hockey player had "had a smile on his face every day." And according to television footage of some of his last moments on ice, he skated pretty fast, too.

I had no inkling my friend Val was depressed until she told me. In Val's case (and mine), we could walk briskly and talk fast and we both smiled a lot. In fact, at my first session, Dr. Menchions noted that I "can 'put on a front' professionally." In the depths of my depressive episode, I even discovered I could look sparklingly happy—with the skilled help of a makeup artist and a talented photographer.

As my new book on Beijing was about to hit the shelves, Indigo, Canada's largest bookstore chain, invited me to take part in its fall marketing campaign. Of course, they didn't know I'd been on Cipralex for four weeks, and was listless and anxious, or that I was beyond caring what I looked like. I knew I should cooperate, but I didn't have the energy to drag myself to the hairdresser. Instead, on a sweltering August day, I showed up at the photographer's loft studio wearing an old T-shirt, khaki shorts and flip-flops. George Whiteside, one of Canada's top fashion and art photographers, greeted me with a glass of chilled mineral water. If he was dismayed by my scruffy appearance, he kept it to himself.

His studio had polished concrete floors, all-white furnishings, and factory-style windows that let in soft northern light. The only splashes of color were a wall of art books and several tabletop collections of *objets*, all arranged by hue (including the books). I took a sip of the mineral water and thoughtlessly set the glass down on his dining table, a polished, fifteen-foot slab of exotic wood. Whiteside snatched it up before it could leave a ruinous ring on the surface. As he swabbed the moisture, I was filled with self-loathing. I didn't belong there. I just wanted to go home to bed.

The makeup artist, a hip young woman dressed all in black, gently suggested I swap my sweaty T-shirt for the pressed magenta blouse I had brought in reserve. As she twirled and ironed my ragged hair into a sleek coif, she chatted amiably about the hot weather. While she applied powder and lipstick and mascara, she dished on all the misbehaving celebrities with whom she had worked. I began to relax.

Then Whiteside posed me on a stool and told me to smile. I tried. I moved the muscles around my mouth. I bared my teeth. I clamped my lips together and curved them upward. I looked stricken. I looked weird. I looked grotesque. I was a complete failure, someone who couldn't even muster a fake smile.

In the midst of his depression, William Styron had to pose for a magazine photographer. "Of the session I can recall little except the first snowflakes of winter dotting the air outside. I thought I obeyed the photographer's request to smile often. A day or two later the magazine's editor telephoned my wife, asking if I would submit to another session. The reason he advanced was that the pictures of me, even the ones with smiles, were 'too full of anguish.'"

Styron didn't have a helpful makeup artist to cajole him past the anguish. Mine planted herself beside the camera lens and began talking and laughing. By then I liked her very much and could smile easily. As I relaxed, Whiteside kept snapping. Within an hour, he had captured enough usable shots for the marketing campaign. I watched as he touched up my image on his computer, swishing away white hairs and erasing wrinkles. He left in a smidgen of crow's feet—"just a bit," he said—so I wouldn't look "plastic." It was a wrap.

The glam photo soon appeared everywhere (and I bought a shot for the back cover of this book, just so you can see the results.) It went up on bus shelters, in subway cars and—this is true—in ads in *The Globe and Mail*. They loomed billboard-size outside and inside Indigo bookstores. I was on the chain's free bookmarks, too, thumbprint-size and beaming. I looked young, pretty and very, very happy.

My psychiatrist noticed the photo and even he assumed it had been taken before I got sick. I would board a subway car and realize the photo filled every single advertising slot. I would look around expectantly, but no one did a double take. Once I was with a friend who was unable to believe that no one was making the connection. She poked the passenger next to her and demanded, "Don't you think that photo looks like her?" Startled, the woman looked up at the advertising strip and then back at me.

"Yes," she nodded. "It looks like you."

I could tell she saw zero resemblance. (I was back to my scruffy self.) I could also tell she thought my friend and I were both loons. The photo didn't look like the real me at all. Which just proved to me that you could be dying inside and still look fabulous, especially if you had the world's nicest makeup artist and a stellar photographer to assist you. The makeover made me feel terrific for a week—until the day of my first mediation.

All I wanted was to regain my health and return to work. Instead, after three months without sick pay, I attended my first mediation. Not knowing what to expect, I was quivering with anxiety. Mediation, I discovered, is a formal, costly process. It involves hiring a trained mediator, renting a special hearing room and, of course, each side paying for its lawyers. Any settlement is voluntary on the part of both parties and almost always confidential. If nothing is resolved, everyone proceeds to arbitration, a high-risk, quasi-judicial process in which the arbitrator's decision is both binding and public.

The *Globe* sent an overwhelming force—editors, lawyers, HR specialists and senior executives. The union sent a lawyer. Norman couldn't come that morning, so Colleen accompanied me instead. During the awkward chitchat before the mediation started, management discovered Colleen and I were heading to Paris the next week.

Suddenly everyone looked furious. Not only was my smiling mug plastered all over the city, I was now flying off for foie gras. That anger and suspicion set the mood for the rest of the day. Mediation is always confidential, so I can't provide details of what happened. All I can say is negotiations quickly deteriorated. The company made an offer I couldn't live with and the union looked hopeful, but I shook my head. I felt frustrated and bereft. After nine hours, the union's lawyer agreed with me. "I can't recommend that you sign this deal," he said, wearily shaking his head.

I left the mediation center, feeling as though I was drowning in an ocean, locked in a life-and-death struggle with a man-eating shark. What I couldn't see is that all the while a tsunami was rolling in. My life was imploding, but I still naively believed I could return to work once I got better. I was trying so hard to make everyone understand I was sick that I only half-heard the roar of the approaching tidal wave.

Perhaps I *was* insane. I should have been worried about my job, but I suppose I was confident these particular executives would all be gone, sooner or later. In the nearly two decades I'd worked at the *Globe*, a dozen editors-in-chief and managing editors had been fired, pushed out or demoted. Whenever a top editor was particularly venal, I would shore up the morale of my fellow reporters by reminding them that our newspaper was like a furnished apartment. We were the wall-to-wall carpet and the managers were the tenants. They walked all over us, but in the end, the lease would expire and they would all move out. We stayed. It was *our* newspaper.

Dr. Menchions anticipated that I would be distraught after mediation and had scheduled an appointment for the next day. When I told him about the hostile reaction to my Paris trip, he sat down at his computer. Typing rapidly for a minute, he wrote that he was "specifically encouraging" me to go. As medical benefits, he cited the "respite" from the situation and said it was a chance for me to "recuperate" from the "high level of anxiety" the situation was causing. "Were she physically disabled," he wrote, "the structure of modified work might provide the same benefits, but since her work is so all-consuming, and the medical issues have to do with her emotions and cognition, then the time away will provide the therapeutic benefit she needs."

That was far too much jargon for me. All I knew was that I was in fight-or-flight mode. And since I couldn't whack my employer, I had to flee. I had to get out of Dodge. At the time, it didn't occur to me that my doctor had been compelled to spell out the nature of depression: "emotions and cognition." He'd had to defend the treatment: "time away will provide the therapeutic benefit." If I had had a brain tumor, he would not have had to explain why I couldn't work. He would not have had to explain what radiation would accomplish. It highlighted to me the big difference in attitude toward mental disabilities and physical ones.

A few days later, Colleen and I flew to Paris. My friend Robert, a Canadian journalist at Agence France Presse, met us in a café to hand over the keys to the apartment of his generous Australian colleague. It was located in Montmartre on rue des Abbesses, an unusually quiet pedestrian lane accessible only by steep, cobblestoned steps. Robert warned us that the nineteenth-century stone building had no front-entrance buzzer. Visitors had to toss a pebble at our fifth-floor window or—the twenty-first-century equivalent—call from a cellphone.

After we dropped off our suitcases, my friend took us on a walking tour. He led us past the gleaming white dome of Sacre-Coeur, the basilica that dominates Paris. He pointed out the *ateliers* of Modigliani, Pissarro and Van Gogh and showed us the little café featured in the hit film *Amélie*. At lunch we stopped at a local café for grilled lamb chops and a carafe of sturdy red wine.

On the second day, my fifty-fifth birthday, my literary agent called with good news. He had found an American publisher for my new Beijing book. Other deals were pending in France, Italy, the Netherlands and Australia. The money would more than cushion my sick-pay stoppage. To celebrate, I treated Colleen to lunch at Atélier Joël Robuchon, a Michelin-starred black-and-red *boîte* on rue de Montalembert. We sat on bar stools at a polished counter, which encircled an open kitchen, lit as dramatically as an opera set. While we sipped apéritifs, we watched the chefs perform their artistry. Our twelve-course tasting menu included scrambled eggs with *girolles* and fresh cream; chilled gazpacho; lobster carpaccio; foie gras with peach-and-hibiscus sauce; sea bass; quail stuffed with more foie gras; and caramelized, truffled potatoes. For dessert, we shared a chocolate *ganache*; some spiced red fruits, and sorbets of verbena, basil and lavender.

Paris was just what the doctor ordered. Colleen and I could walk downhill from Montmartre to Opéra and Galéries Lafayette. Or we could jump on the Métro, and arrive fifteen minutes later at the Louvre. Our borrowed three-bedroom apartment was unusually spacious by Parisian standards. Across the narrow street, we had stunning views of St.-Jean-de-Montmartre Church whose magnificent bells chimed reliably every hour and, to my delight, occasionally played fragments of Bach. Each morning, I slept until the slanting sun awoke me. Colleen, bless her, rose early, walked down five flights of stairs, up the steep steps of rue des Abbesses and down again to rue Lépic where the nearby shops were just pulling up their shutters. She brought back buttery croissants, *pain au chocolat*, crisp baguettes, artisanal butter, runny cheeses, organic eggs and raspberry *confiture*. My biggest concern each day was not ruining my appetite for lunch.

It was such a relief to put actual distance between my stressor and myself, and yet, at the same time, I remained deeply depressed. I was no longer weeping constantly, but I could not out-travel my sadness. Alas, after ten days, Colleen had to get back to her job. Because the prospect of being alone frightened me, Ben had volunteered to stay with me for the last week.

He had already seen the sights six years earlier during a family vacation, so we took it easy. We listened to sidewalk musicians on the Left Bank and watched daredevil rollerbladers in front of Nôtre Dame Cathedral. He window-shopped with me at Fauchon, the luxe grocer in Place de la Madeleine. He patiently accompanied me to E. Dehillerin, at 18 rue Coquillière, supplier of copper pots to French chefs since 1820. Together, we tried the *Vélib*, the newly installed system of public bikes. Shakily, then with growing confidence, I cycled on a sturdy but stylish silver bicycle up and down the busy streets, even taking a cautious spin through Place Vendôme, past the Ritz Hotel. My son was not overly embarrassed to be seen riding a *Vélib* bicycle with his mom.

Ben, who was seventeen by then, would have much preferred hanging out at home with his girlfriend. He had come to Paris only because he knew I was sick. Each day, he thoughtfully asked *me* what I wanted to see or do. One afternoon we spotted a poster advertising a cello concert at Saint-Ephrem, a tiny Romanesque church famous for its acoustics. We grabbed an early dinner of *raclette*, melted cheese eaten with pickles, boiled potatoes and cured beef, and then hurried to the church. Timothée Marcel, a prize-winning graduate of the Paris Conservatory, was performing Bach. Sitting on tiny reed chairs in the front row, we were so close we could hear Marcel breathe in sync with his phrasing. The music, the first and third of Bach's "Six Suites for Unaccompanied Cello", was divine. This time, Ben did not doze off. In fact, he declared it the best concert he had ever attended. I had always wanted to share my love of music with my boys and was ridiculously happy afterward when he bought a copy of the young musician's CD and asked for an autograph.

Ben and I stuffed ourselves every day. We ate couscous *royale*; icy Belon oysters sprinkled with minced shallots and red wine vinegar; *soupe a l'oignon*; steak tartare; *choucroute garnie*; breaded and grilled pig's feet; *lapin à la moutarde*; *pain perdu* with artisanal coffee ice cream; *frisée aux lardons*; more foie gras; duck *confit*; crepes with chestnut cream; sidewalk falafel; and roasted marrow bones sprinkled with *fleur de sel*. When we passed a *patisserie*, which seemed to happen every ten minutes, we bought treats that we devoured right then on the sidewalk: sugar-dusted Chantilly cream puffs the size of softballs, *tartlettes* of red currants and handfuls of crisp raspberry and pistachio macarons. Near our apartment, on rue Blanche,

I discovered Domaine de Lintillac, a duck restaurant run by an agricultural cooperative. A couple at a neighboring table advised me to order the *specialité*, a bargain-priced duck breast grilled in its own unctuous fat, served sliced and ruby rare, with potatoes fried in garlic and more duck fat. An accompanying glass of sweet, golden Monbazillac completed the feast.

Don't hate me. During my trip, I didn't gain weight. Depression meant I could eat all the time and my system would barely absorb the calories. I was "failing to thrive," though such failure was pretty damn wonderful in Paris.

Away from the stressors of daily life, I did not try to throw Ben's laptop out the fifth-floor window onto the cobblestones of rue des Abbesses. I had made some progress since my hockey trip to Finland and did not feel the need to cling to my children every moment. I began to forge a new, healthier relationship with my seventeen year old. In the evening I let him explore the city alone and he would return refreshed and excited. The next day we would both sleep in and then eat a gargantuan lunch at a sidewalk café, sometimes in companionable silence, sometimes discussing the French Revolution or sneaking glances at a giddy wedding party at the next table. It occurred to me that a parent-child relationship is the only love relationship where one side's goal is to ensure the other side eventually leaves. In my illness I had neglected my children, but somehow that same illness brought my sons closer to me. My teenagers had rallied to my side and supported me through it all. Being with Ben in Paris, just the two of us, was one of the gifts of my depression. Had I not been depressed, I doubt that he would have deigned to spend an entire week alone with me that summer. But he did. My troubles did not go away, but we had fun. We *both* had fun. It was the upside of being down.

PART IV

HEALING

CHAPTER 19

Fight or Flight?

I lied. I gained three pounds in Paris. Alas, upon my return I found myself sinking deeper into despair. The company and the union had jointly chosen an arbitrator who was so heavily booked she would not be able to hear my case for another *year*. I was devastated. Was this a ploy by both sides to force me to take the initial offer? I knew the long delay would prolong my depression. Certainly, it meant many more months without pay.

By now there were so many mediations I began to lose track. There were separate hearings to settle disputes between management and the union over sick pay, reprimands and insurance forms. Belatedly I discovered I also had to attend a separate mediation over the disciplinary letters in my personnel file. Within days, I shed my three Parisian pounds. My blood pressure went off the charts. "You're too stressed," said Dr. Au, who was trying to measure it. "Pretend you're sitting on the beach." I took a deep breath and closed my eyes. I felt the sand between my toes. I could hear the surf. Magically, my blood pressure dropped to normal. There it was—the direct link between mind and body.

At the mediation over the disciplinary letters, we met for five hours and got nowhere. The mediator shuttled impotently back and forth between two windowless conference rooms. Then we all went home. As the conflict deepened, each side was bloodied. My losses included my health, sanity and income. Theirs included a once-productive employee, management time and energy, and even more money. By late 2007, I estimated the company had already spent fifty thousand dollars on legal fees alone, about what it owed me in sick pay.

Outsiders were mystified. "Who cares what the fight is about? You brought in readers. Now they've helped destroy a key asset. It makes no sense," said a retired CEO and board member on a rival newspaper. Others craved a logical explanation. They kept asking why my company persisted when I had all the medical paperwork. I think they wanted to understand just in case they ever had to dodge a similar bullet themselves. I had no sure answers. Perhaps companies try to purge those with depression for fear the condition becomes chronic. There is, after all, that 50-percent chance of relapse. Or perhaps management tries to make an example of anyone who pushes back. My treatment brought to mind a Chinese aphorism: "Kill the chicken to scare the monkeys."

I wonder now whether other problems at work were setting me up for a breakdown long before it actually happened. Like so many people in other industries, I had been under pressure to produce more in less time. My own ambition fueled this; I *wanted* to work flat out. Ironically, my history as a workaholic may have even made management suspicious. Why, all of a sudden, was I unable to write? I had always churned out the goods before.

The ancient fight-or-flight response must be hard-wired in us. The second I got back from Paris, I wanted to flee again. I began amassing travel brochures. I studied airfares in the windows of discount travel agencies. I surfed the Internet for getaway deals. I fantasized about trips to Egypt, Spain, Zimbabwe. Then my literary agent suggested I meet with my New York publisher. *That* I couldn't do—what if I broke down in tears? I didn't want them to think they'd just bought a book from a crazy woman.

Still, once I began thinking about New York, I couldn't stop. It was one hour away by plane. I loved the city. And I could camp on my niece's dorm-room floor at Columbia University. I asked my psychiatrist what he thought. "Paris helped you," he said. "So this might, too."

I flew to New York. To my surprise, in the quarter-century since I'd left Columbia, the washrooms had become distressingly co-ed, without even a private nook to change for a shower. Shielded only by a small towel, I had to hop naked back and forth across the hall. I didn't know whether to feel relieved—or even more depressed—when no one gave me a second glance.

At a newsstand, I bought a copy of the *New Yorker* to check the entertainment listings. A brief item about Kathleen Battle caught my eye. Thirteen years earlier, Joseph Volpe, the general manager of the Metropolitan Opera, had fired her from the starring role in *La Fille du Régiment*. A *New York Times* article accused the soprano of behaving— surprise—like a diva. Battle was forty-five when she was fired. She never sang an opera role again.

Then Peter Gelb, a friend of Battle's, became the Met's new general manager. He suggested she return to the opera house, but the soprano declined. "She told me that for ten years, every time she walked down Broadway, she crossed to the other side of the street rather than set foot on Lincoln Center property," he told the *New Yorker*.

I understood. At home, I had to avert my eyes whenever I passed *Globe* boxes on the sidewalk. For more than a year, I could not go near the company's headquarters on Front Street. When I spied it from the Gardiner Expressway, out of the corner of my eye, I had to look away. Even now, it pains me when friends and neighbors mention that they have read something interesting in the *Globe*. If they notice the expression on my face, they apologize awkwardly, as if they have blurted out the name of an ex-boyfriend.

Joan Didion calls this "the vortex effect." In the year after her husband, John Gregory Dunne, died of a heart attack, she would avoid certain streets, restaurants, even entire cities. "I plotted my routes, I remained on guard." Sometimes, it would not be a place but a date that would trigger a cascade of traumatic memories. On the first anniversary of their daughter's wedding, she suddenly found herself in tears when she remembered her husband asking which tie he should wear to the church. Something insignificant had, following a great loss, become an excruciating memory.

Thinking about Kathleen Battle, I stopped by the Metropolitan Opera House. The only remaining ticket for the next day's performance of *Madama Butterfly* cost a breathtaking $320. Like the overpriced cocktail dress I felt I had needed as armor, I thought: I *need* Puccini. I plunked down my Visa card, and then walked across the plaza to Avery Fisher Hall and bought a $45 ticket to the London Symphony Orchestra for the night after. Or I thought I did. Blame the meds or depression, or both. I had, in fact, just bought non-refundable, non-exchangeable tickets for two concerts on the same night.

Somehow spending money, even stupidly on same-night tickets, alleviated my gloom. I bought an armful of books from Barnes & Noble, an ergonomically correct tomato peeler (even though I never peel tomatoes), some good French wine for Norman, a box of Belgian chocolates for the boys, Jockey brand undershirts and blue jeans for myself. Across from the cratered remains of the twin towers, I prowled through Century 21, a discount-designer department store, and found an outrageous pink-and-red flowered, sequined sweater-jacket of Italian cashmere and silk. At Bloomingdales, I snapped up a slinky, black, floor-length Anne Klein dress.

Back in my niece's dorm after an exhilarating day of shopping, I suddenly remembered that Melvin Mencher, my favorite journalism teacher, lived three blocks away. "Come on over," he said, when I phoned. The professor lived a five-minute walk from campus in a spacious, university-owned apartment overlooking the Hudson River. When he opened the door, I was struck by how he little he had changed. His thick mane of hair had gone from jet black to pure white, but he was still barrel-chested, with piercing blue eyes and expressive, balletic hands.

Seeing the professor reminded me that New York was where I had launched myself into journalism, where I had learned the craft. *Put good quotes up high. Question authority. There's no such thing as a stupid question.* Professor Mencher had taught me the rules of journalism, and then he taught me how to break them, too. What he really taught me was truth-telling and storytelling. It had been twenty-six years since I had graduated, but I was one of many students who had kept in touch with him over the decades.

He handed me a mug of milky tea and settled into his armchair. He listened intently while I told him about the school shooting, the backlash and my depression. "The business is in decline," he said in his distinctive gravelly voice. "It's struggling. The last thing they want is what we used to call a 'shit disturber.' They want a placid, easygoing reporter. They don't want *you*.... You're like the sand in the oyster. Bland is in. Twelve words per sentence. Three graphs per story."

I winced. No one had summed it up for me quite so bluntly. For the first time, I began to feel uneasy about the possibility, or rather, the impossibility of going back to the newsroom. Was my professor right? My industry *was* changing. Newspapers had once prized reporters with courage and persistence. Management once promoted those who dared to stand up to authority. But those qualities weren't in demand any more. They certainly weren't welcome *inside* the workplace. As my professor pointed out, management preferred obedience and compliance. They didn't want someone who read an insurance form before signing it.

Melvin Mencher had worked just twelve years as a reporter. Then he had written a story about young widows, how they missed the intimacies of daily life with a partner. They missed brushing their teeth in the morning with someone beside them. An editor had cut that detail and it broke Mencher's heart. He quit, and got a job teaching journalism at the University of Kansas. There he heard a rumor that the administration maintained racially segregated lists of off-campus housing. He sent his students to check it out. In a classic investigative maneuver, first the white students obtained the addresses of vacant apartments. Then black students tried to rent them. Every single apartment—surprise—was already rented. Then of course the white students went back to the same apartments. Miraculously they had become available again. The article made a splash and annoyed the local pillars of society. The dean called in Mencher for a chat that didn't end well. But Columbia University picked him up, a gig that lasted thirty-two years, until it soured, too. He took a buy-out in 1990, when he was sixty-one.

"In a way it's all my fault," he mused. "All my students have trouble. What else is journalism about? It's the obligatory response of journalists to question authority."

He checked his watch. We had already been talking for two hours. He suggested we get some lunch at a Cuban restaurant on Broadway, across from the red-brick journalism building at Columbia. Over chicken and rice and beans, I told him I loved my job and wanted to go back. I said that it was all I ever wanted.

"You're a workaholic," he said dismissively. "You're afraid of losing journalism. A lot of reporters are like dope addicts. They want the quick payoff from writing. The creative act is very pleasurable. It's a satisfying act, almost like sex itself."

He was right. The chase. The scoop. The instant gratification. This was what had made me stay all night on my hotel balcony as the bullets flew at Tiananmen Square. It was what had sent me racing to New York City the day after 9/11. I *was* addicted. I didn't want to quit.

"Forget it," he growled. "It's over. IT. IS. OVER. Three words. Subject. Verb. Object. You know they don't want you. You're an irritant."

I felt the tears brimming in my eyes. I wasn't ready to quit and I told him that. He pushed away his plate and continued his lecture-for-one. "In the past, you've been prized for being a pain in the ass. You've lost. You're a loser. We're all losers. They need us, but they don't want us. Unfortunately, you're not crazy. You're just dispirited. Unhappy. You thrive in battle. You're what is known in the trade as a tough cookie. The question is: will you continue to thrive on conflict? No, because you're breaking down. *Move on.* That's got to become your mantra."

How could I move on? Daily journalism was my core. My job wasn't just a paycheck (even if I wasn't getting one any more). It was a job where you stamped your byline on the finished product for everyone to see. If I stopped being a reporter, then who was I? Losing it would feel like a near-death experience.

Professor Mencher and I had been talking for five hours. He stared at me from across the table. "You fought as a student. You fought me. And you were absolutely right."

I couldn't believe he remembered. In 1981, a fellow student and I had teamed up to write an investigative piece on New York taxis. He had given an A to me, but only a C to her. My classmate was devastated. I told her to sit tight. Then I marched into the professor's office and told him he was wrong to give us different marks because we had contributed equally to the project. And by the way, I added, I wasn't going to accept a C. He raised my partner's mark to an A.

Now I looked at my old professor for final words of guidance. He sighed. "Do you go back or do you change your life?" he asked. It was a question he would not answer for me. "You don't want to confront it because it's too great a loss. It's what you love."

I tried to give away the surplus symphony ticket. My niece was too busy. So was a group of students rehearsing chamber music in the main-floor common room. I spied a young Asian man walking down Broadway, carrying a violin case. When I tried to give him the ticket, he fled in wordless terror. Professor Mencher couldn't use the ticket either. "Just go down and throw yourself on their mercy."

I'd always followed his advice. That evening, I went back to the box office at Avery Fisher Hall. As I waited in line, I overheard the woman in front of me tell her friend that they needed just one ticket to the London Symphony Orchestra. Unfortunately, she added, the concert was sold out. I tapped her on the shoulder. "I have a ticket."

"Will you sell it to me?" she asked eagerly, turning around.

Suddenly the clerks behind the wickets started shouting. One of them rapped the window with her ring. "You can't sell tickets in here!" she yelled. Another clerk shouted, "It's illegal to sell tickets!" A security guard rushed over. My shoulders slumped as I prepared to be arrested. My eyes filled with tears. My hands shook. The woman who wanted my ticket took charge. "Come outside," she said calmly. "We can talk outside."

On the festively lit plaza of Lincoln Center, we completed our contraband deal. Still trembling, I took my seat inside the Metropolitan Opera House. When the house lights dimmed, I had a little cry. On stage, Butterfly was weeping bitterly. If those around me noticed my damp cheeks, I hoped they would assume I was just another crazy opera buff. I was, in fact, just crazy.

Smile, You're on Candid Camera

I was trying to describe yet another symptom to my psychiatrist: the intermittent twitch under my left eye. "It's like something crazy people have."

"It's not *crazy*," Dr. Menchions said testily. He hated when I used that word. Then he suddenly said, "I want you to think of life without *The Globe and Mail*."

"You mean I should quit?" I asked, startled.

"No, I just mean that you should start *thinking* about doing other things. Try to imagine yourself doing something else."

It was another of the doctor's well-timed nudges. I told him my professor at Columbia had just told me the same thing. In twenty years I had never considered leaving the *Globe*, not even when other newspapers and magazines had tried to lure me away. My psychiatrist didn't say another word. He just kept staring at me. After a long moment, I gulped and told him yes, I would try to start imagining a new life.

My immediate problem was the upcoming book tour for *Beijing Confidential*.

Was I up to it? In fact, I could hardly wait. A book tour was the essence of escape, every day a literal flight to a different city, a new hotel. From past tours, I knew the interviewers typically asked soft questions. Friendly folk would plunk down good money for my book. Some might even ask me to sign it. What could be more therapeutic? This book tour was scheduled to take me to seven cities across Canada. Escorts would meet me at airports and drive me to appointments. All I had to do was bathe regularly. Oh, and talk endlessly about myself. That I could certainly do.

As usual, my psychiatrist was unequivocal. "The book tour is rehabilitative," he said. "It will help bring you back into your old world, without the stresses of your job. You're very fragile right now. Your memory is not functioning. You are doing no creative writing at moment. There is no partial recovery with your situation."

This was my doctor's blunt opinion, but I worried about how the *Globe* would react. How dare I go on a book tour if I was too disabled to work?

I scoured my conscience. I considered my continuing inability to write. I had written *Beijing Confidential* during the book leave the *Globe* itself had pressed me to take. Then I'd had the relapse after receiving fresh hate emails, after management accused me of cooperating with the writer of the *Toronto Life* article (and put a new letter in my personnel file), after my feature on Conrad Black had been mysteriously spiked. Now, following my brief return to the newsroom, I couldn't even manage to write a letter. I had trouble remembering appointments, I suffered from insomnia, I still cried with annoying frequency. I asked myself: was a book tour a form of journalism? Would I have to interview anyone or report any stories? No, I would not. A book tour was a celebration of my accomplishments as an author. At the nadir of my professional life, I knew that if I didn't go on tour, my depression would worsen. Every other part of my career was in ashes.

I knew by now that Manulife frowned on travel of any sort. Not that it mattered; my intervention specialist appeared to have severed all contact with me following my relapse and the withholding of my sick pay. At the same time, I had reached the point where I had stopped trying to convince my employer that I *was* sick. No matter what medical reports and doctors' notes I provided, the company didn't believe me. And it was still refusing to talk to either my family doctor or my psychiatrist. I couldn't put my recovery on hold until management came around. I now knew it was important to escape from the stressors. To get better, I had to go out and do the things I loved.

Andrew Solomon also was determined to go on a book tour in the middle of one of his three breakdowns. "I knew that the more I managed to do, the less I would want to die, so it seemed important to go." That was how I felt— it seemed important to go. By appearing on radio and television, it might look like I was committing journalism. But as every journalist knows, the difference between interviewing someone and being interviewed is like the difference between performing surgery and undergoing it.

My chief fear was fielding questions about the *Globe*. I wasn't even allowed to say that I wasn't allowed to talk. I told my psychiatrist that I needed a script. "Speak in generalities about the ups and downs of the business. Say, 'In our business...' Focus on the book. Don't talk about personal circumstances. It's not helpful on the book tour to talk about being sick."

It seemed simple enough, but it felt anything but simple. What if the interviewer pressed me? I worried about follow-up questions. What if I broke down on live television? I must have looked stricken.

"You see—the very fact that you're asking me what to say means you're not better," he said. "Normally, you wouldn't need to ask anyone."

I nodded glumly and told him the Celexa wasn't working. He suggested another antidepressant. But I didn't want to risk starting a new drug while on the tour. So he doubled my dosage and gave me his pager number for emergencies.

Much later I read his clinical notes:

- *ready for tour (I reiterate how she can benefit from the structure without the demands of the investigative journalism she is so good at when well.)*
- *worried about tour—almost has a guilt-driven sense that it's "wrong" to do it if cannot work.*
- *reiterate to her that her own job involves: focus, drive, persistence, quick-wittedness, curiosity and stamina which she doesn't have now, but that she needs to try to re-connect as best as she can to 'world.'*
- *Wonders what to say if asked about Dawson College. Normally, she wouldn't be seeking counsel on that at all*
- *GAF score 55-60 "well below her normal"*
  Continue meds.

By going on my book tour, I was inadvertently walking into an epic insurance fight. In the 1980s, faced with soaring claims for mental disability, Canadian insurers had collectively and unilaterally attempted to cap payments at twenty-four months. But in 1996 the Supreme Court of Canada struck down that industry-wide pact. The highest court called it discriminatory because there was no similar cap on physical-disability payments. It ordered insurance companies to treat mental and physical disabilities the same.

A psychiatrist named Erhard Busse told *Benefits Canada*, a trade publication, that the Supreme Court ruling had changed the economic landscape. No longer able to limit psychiatric claims to two years, companies now faced an unlimited drain on the bottom line. "The economic impact on insurance companies and the workplace has been huge," said Dr. Busse, then head of a consulting company handling disability claims for employers and insurers. Of all the mental-disability claims he had personally reviewed, 80 percent were linked to unresolved workplace problems. Therefore he urged insurers to set up early-intervention programs and effective return-to-work strategies. Otherwise, he warned, a mental illness could evolve into a long-term disability case. "You want to get to people while they are still open to choices. In three to six months, they get locked into the lifestyle of the disabled," said Busse.

He also warned about the consequences of pushing people too hard. "It's easy to bully people back to work only to have them crash within a month. That's not what you want to do." Certainly, I had "crashed" after six weeks back at work. This time, the second time around, I was much more cautious. I didn't want another relapse. This time I was determined to do everything my psychiatrist recommended. If he thought a book tour was rehabilitative, then I would go.

With the book tour about to begin, I expected the Manulife intervention specialist to call, and she did. She hadn't been in touch for nearly a year, not since the previous Christmas when my sick pay had been stopped the first time. But she picked up just where we left off.

"When we last talked, you were still upset and angry," she said. "Do you remember?"

I said nothing.

"You probably don't, if you're having memory problems."

She said that I was mere days away from moving out of STD, or short-term disability, to LTD, or long-term disability. As Manulife was responsible for paying LTD, she announced that the insurer was about to start sending me monthly tax-free checks.

My heart leapt.

"To process this claim," she added, "I need to get medical records."

My heart sank.

More paperwork. More records. More reports. Every time I had to sort through my files and revisit the chronology, my anxiety and depression would deepen. It was perplexing. Three health professionals, including one of theirs, had already advised them I was sick. Both my doctors had already provided extensive notes and diagnostic reports. What more did they want? In fact, what Manulife now wanted was *all* of my psychiatrist's clinical notes from every single session *and* a record of every psychiatric appointment I had ever attended *and* a list of all my medications. I felt myself get sicker, but I told the intervention specialist I would try to pull that together for her.

"I'm noticing you sound much more in control, much calmer," she said warmly. "You sound *much* better."

Again, I said nothing.

Then she came to the point. The intervention specialist said that she had heard I was going on a book tour. The tour wasn't a secret—it was, after all, a *publicity* tour—but I didn't know how to say that without sounding rude. At any rate, she didn't give me a chance to speak. She said that from the *Globe's* perspective, my book tour was work. If Manulife's legal department agreed, this would disqualify me for those monthly tax-free disability checks she had just mentioned, the ones that were supposed to start arriving any day now.

I began to tremble. It seemed pointless to debate with her the practical differences between working as a journalist and touring as an author. But this seemed as good an opportunity as any to ask a question. I had wondered for some time whether my employer had ever been informed about the recommendations in the independent medical exam. Specifically, I wondered if anyone had read the report's last page. The intervention specialist didn't seem to know what I was talking about, so I retrieved the report from my desk drawer and read aloud:

Ms. Wong appears motivated to return to work at this time. I suggest in the interest of facilitating a productive and sustainable work return that this be done with the utmost consideration to her emotional wellbeing and while being mindful of the fact that her condition is in partial remission at this time.

The intervention specialist sounded surprised. Then she acknowledged that she had never passed on the report from the independent psychiatrist. That meant that no one had told the *Globe* that I was not fully recovered.

"Next time we'll get your doctor to write to them," the intervention specialist promised.

Next time. This was already my second time around. Was there going to be a third round? And what good would another doctor's report do?

"As we move forward, let's not make the same mistakes." She sighed. "You're a reporter. You should do a story on it."

My union was dubious about the book tour, too. The rep warned me that my doctor would have to testify. He emailed me saying: "I remember a case at the [Toronto] *Star* when a member on stress leave met up with a manager while playing shinny at the local rink!"

That exclamation mark said it all. Like so many of us, the union rep did not understand mental disability. How can you skate and push around a little black vulcanized rubber puck, yet be too disabled to work? *Gotcha!* Or, speaking of hockey players, how could someone grin for the television cameras while learning to ice dance with a figure skater and then go back to his condo and hang himself? *Gotcha!*

Or smile on the beach? *Gotcha!*

In 2009, Manulife Financial cut off long-term disability benefits to a twenty-nine-year-old IBM employee in Quebec who had been off work for depression. The insurer discovered Facebook photos of her on a beach. She told reporters that her doctor had advised her to travel. Perhaps the geographic cure was working! She was *smiling!* The story was news because it was one of the first times an insurer had investigated a claimant using social-network information. But what struck me was how depression and one of its cures—escaping particular stressors—is so misunderstood. The ancient fight-or-flight reflex is misconstrued as latter-day fraud.

Worse, many employers and insurers specifically prohibit the geographic cure. A friend who works in human resources said that her company, a major media conglomerate in Toronto, bars people on disability from leaving the province of Ontario. When her company recently refused to allow a depressed employee to visit his family in Newfoundland, he quit. My *Globe* colleague, the one who had several relapses, told me that she had yearned to spend her final week of sick leave recharging at a beach resort. Her Manulife intervention specialist told her that was not allowed. My colleague obediently stayed in Toronto, returned to work and soon fell apart.

When I first began traveling on my doctor's advice, I hadn't realized it was an insurance no-no. And after I knew it was forbidden, well, I had already been cut off from my disability benefits. Perhaps it's understandable that those working in human resources tend to see travel as proof of robust health. They're not medical experts. Why should they be better informed than the rest of the populace? But insurers, who hire psychologists and psychiatrists and other expert consultants, do know better. And if they don't, they damn well ought to. Disability is their business. Instead, they cynically take advantage of the age-old prejudice against mental illness to avoid paying disability. A century ago, no one could see cancer tumors either. Were people with cancer treated as slackers when they didn't spring out of bed and saddle up the horse?

I began the tour with a book launch at the trendy Gladstone Hotel in Toronto. I recall almost nothing about it, only that it was raining hard that night and I wore a fuchsia silk gown. My friend, Paul, remembers I was brimming with insecurity. "Because you hadn't been writing for the *Globe* for so long, you had lost your identity. You had self-doubt about whether people would remember who you were."

Apparently, I got Paul so worried no one would show up, he came in the torrential downpour, dragging along his pregnant wife, Isabel. "We thought we'd fill a couple of seats. But the place was overflowing and we had to stand at the back. You ran out of books to sign."

Later, when I saw a video recording of the event, I was amazed to see so many colleagues there from the *Globe*. Had I been so wrong about them? Had I misremembered the silence, the lack of support from workplace friends? Had they in fact reached out to me and I simply had not understood? The video shows that many *Globe* friends and other journalists came to the launch, bought my book and lined up for my autograph. (Colleagues! Asking for my autograph!) It was more evidence of how depression affects a person's perception of reality. I had thought no one cared.

With my memory such a problem, my performance on the book tour was precarious. I sometimes lost my place in the middle of a speech. Once, on live television, I couldn't remember what city I was in. Several interviewers asked about the *Globe*. Then my eyes would fill with tears and my voice would quaver.

In Montreal, I remained fearful someone might try to kill me. I asked a radio station there that had heavily promoted my appearance to let me in through the back door. (They told me to use the front door and not to worry.) When I posed on the sidewalk for a newspaper photo, I kept an eye out for the gunman. The inside of my left cheek became badly swollen from accidental chomping. My left eye still twitched and now so did a muscle just above my right knee. I kept my psychiatrist's pager number tucked, like a talisman, in my purse.

By chance, the tour brought me to Montreal on the anniversary of Mom's passing. Chinese traditionally commemorate a loved one by bowing three times at the gravesite and offerings plates of dim sum. But Mom had been cremated so there was no grave. What's more, our family had been in Canada for more than a century and we weren't well versed in the old rituals. So in an unorthodox twist, we decided to take Mom's ashes with us to dinner instead. In the bustling Chinatown restaurant, Gigi, Dad and I sat down and ordered steamed fish, crispy chicken and sautéed bok choy. Keeping my voice low so as not to alarm the waiters, I addressed the polished wood box on the table beside me and updated Mom on what the grandchildren were doing. Then I told her that I was having problems at the office.

"I'm not at work right now, Mom," I said softly. "I'm sick. I'm trying to get better."

My mother had been my first fan. She had saved every article I had ever written and had spent hours pasting them in thick scrapbooks. The past year and more would have shocked her. She would have been outraged on my behalf. I think she would have understood my depression, too. Perhaps she might have disclosed more about her own struggle with the illness and been able to give me advice about how to muddle through. Suddenly, I missed her very much.

I have a confession to make. I *did* smile now and then on my book tour. And Manulife was there to record it. To my astonishment, the insurer hired Garda, a security agency best known for safeguarding buildings and hauling bullion, to surreptitiously videotape me. I was so paranoid about snipers it never occurred to me I'd be shot instead with a video camera that secretly recorded my every smile. I would not find out about the surveillance until months later, when my lawyer obtained the DVDs from Manulife.

Here's my advice to Garda: don't relocate to Hollywood.

The recordings were comically amateurish. The videographer didn't always know how to turn on the microphone. Every time I smiled, the camera zoomed in for a close up. When my smile faded, the camera zoomed away for a wide-angle shot. It was like that 1960s show, "Smile, You're on Candid Camera." The surveillance recordings also reminded me of Communist China in the 1980s. Back then plain-clothes agents would film me using cameras clumsily hidden inside cheap vinyl shoulder bags. When I pulled out *my* camera and snapped photos of *them*, they invariably scattered in panic.

Garda secretly filmed my book launch at Toronto's Gladstone Hotel. (That's how I know so many of my *Globe* colleagues were there.) A Garda agent also filmed a joint lunchtime appearance with my colleague, Christie Blatchford, at the Metro Toronto Reference Library. It filmed a book talk I gave at the Art Gallery of Hamilton and a book signing I did at the Omni Hotel ballroom in Montreal. Garda saved a lot of effort by downloading a YouTube file of my appearance on CBC television's *The Hour*.

These were public appearances, of course, and it was perfectly legal for Garda/Manulife to record them. But the clandestine creepiness of it all unnerves me. The recording that most upset me was a grainy one of me with my father and sister standing on the sidewalk on the anniversary of Mom's death. I guess it was included to show I could stand upright, but it bothered me. Unlike the other recordings of my book tour, Garda had inadvertently captured an intensely private and sad family moment. We were about to go out for dinner with my mother's ashes.

Much later, I studied how I looked from video to video. On the sidewalk, I seemed anxious and drawn. On stage, I sparkled. Kay Redfield Jamison has written about the gap that frequently exists between public image and private despair. "I appear at times merry and in good heart," she writes. "Talk, too, before others quite reasonable ... yet the soul maintains its deathly sleep and the heart bleeds from a thousand wounds."

Manulife sent the four Garda DVDs for assessment to an industry consultant and psychiatrist named ... Erhard Busse. If his name sounds familiar, it's because he's the expert quoted above, who warned that industry profits would plunge after the Supreme Court struck down the two-year cap on mental-disability payments. According to internal Manulife documents obtained by my lawyer, Busse watched two of the Garda DVDs in their entirety, only parts of the third one and none at all of the fourth. He was unable to turn on the sound to any of them. (He and that Garda videographer would make a great team.)

Nevertheless, Busse diagnosed me based on these DVDs, without ever meeting me. Here are some excerpts from the report he filed to Manulife:

> None of the recordings had an audio component that I was able to listen to, however when she approached the stage she walked briskly, there seemed to be no hesitation, when she spoke her hand movements were brisk and precise ... and there appeared to be no long pauses suggesting uncertainty or hesitation ... I was unable to open one of the CDs [sic] but the last CD [sic] I viewed, at least I viewed large cross sections of it, was the one dated 11/11/07. Here she seemed to be at a meet-the-public event where she was speaking freely and vivaciously to numerous people who came up to her. There was no evidence of psychomotor retardation, there was no evidence of hesitation or uncertainty, and there was no facial expression suggesting confusion or doubt ... It is clearly not the picture of a functionally impaired person suffering from a psychiatric disease. I want to repeat once again though that the audio portion was not available to me ... In all of this I see a vivacious, engaged person showing a full range of emotions. That observed behavior would not suggest to me that we are dealing with a serious and limiting psychiatric disease at that time.

I plead guilty to looking vivacious, especially with my weight loss and the snazzy sequined jacket I bought at Century 21 in New York. I smiled. I spoke briskly, mainly so I could answer the question before I forgot what I'd just been asked. I only got lost a few times during my speeches, but that wouldn't matter because Busse couldn't hear what I was saying anyway. Andrew Solomon struggled on his book tour, too. At a public reading, he writes, "I felt as though I had baby powder in my mouth, and I couldn't hear well, and I kept thinking I might faint, but I managed to do it."

My psychiatrist calls this ability of an author to speak during a book tour the "riding-a-bicycle" theory. "You make speeches all the time, so no matter how depressed you are, you're going to get in front of a crowd and know what to do," Dr. Menchions says. "You may lose your spot from time to time, but you can pull it off. It's like a professional athlete. I'm sure lots of them play [while they're] depressed. They might not be as good as usual, but they get on the field and play."

What *does* a depressed person look like? Perhaps like Jim Carrey, with his wide, wide grin. Watching him yuk his way through his latest comedy, you'd never guess he has suffered from severe depression for years. Or take Owen Wilson, the Hollywood funnyman with the crooked nose and blond mop. His eyes twinkle in his movies—but in 2007 he sliced his wrists.

I mentioned Busse's conclusions to Steven J. Stein, a clinical psychologist who plays saxophone in my Monday-night band. He's the author of *Emotional Intelligence for Dummies* and, as CEO of Multi-Health Systems in Toronto, has consulted for the Canadian Forces, the U.S. Air Force, the Pentagon, the FBI, American Express, Air Canada, Canyon Ranch resorts and several professional sports teams. Stein was shocked that a psychiatrist would conclude I wasn't clinically depressed without interviewing me. "If you were a psychologist, you could lose your licence for that," he said, shaking his head. He added that psychologists do view the occasional tape, but protocol requires that the patient always be present so that questions can be asked, including about context.

"We're not trained as spies or private eyes. What does ten minutes tell you out of, say, 22,000 hours of a person's life?" Stein said that a psychologist he knows once evaluated a man based on a video-surveillance recording taken in a bar. The professional licensing board subsequently censured the psychologist.

Psychiatry hews to a different standard. There is no rule barring psychiatrists from assessing people without meeting them. This practice does, however, elicit ridicule. In 1996 Vivian Rakoff, a professor emeritus at the University of Toronto's department of psychiatry, was mocked for reading some speeches and an autobiography of Quebec premier Lucien Bouchard and then concluding he was "vain," "narcissistic" and suffering from a "character disorder."

Most psychiatrists believe that depression can be verified only through a patient's self-report. To figure out whether an antidepressant drug is working, for instance, you must ask the person taking it. This leaves the door open to abuse—by both sides. An insurer can rule that a secretly videotaped patient looks "vivacious" and deny the claim for disability. Claimants can abuse the system, too.

Stein told me he occasionally administers tests to catch fraudulent claims of mental illness. I was intrigued. What if someone knew enough to fake typical symptoms, say, sleeplessness, crying and forgetfulness?

"We will catch them," Stein said.

"How?"

He didn't want to give away trade secrets, but I pressed for an example. Finally he said, "We'll ask a question about dizziness, which isn't a typical symptom of depression, to try to catch the person out."

I asked the same question of my psychiatrist, who sometimes also assesses employees on behalf of employers. Can you fake depression? "You could fake it really well, but it would be easy to catch if you had just textbook knowledge." Given enough rope, Dr. Menchions says, almost everyone who is faking it slips up after a while. But he adds that many people genuinely experience some stress and anxiety at work.

"A lot of people would never deliberately make up a story. But the unconscious mind is very powerful. There is an unconscious expansion— *somebody owes me something around here.* I would say they're not setting out to scam, but the unconscious mind has made four into eight."

Insurers and employers are right to presume that some people *are* out to scam them. But for genuine sufferers of depression, the bar may be set impossibly high. Dizziness isn't a typical symptom of depression, as my friend, Steven Stein, says. But dizziness *is* a possible side effect of Effexor. And withdrawal symptoms of Celexa also include dizziness.

The lack of an objective test for depression—biochemical, brain scan, what have you—means a fight with insurers is often an inevitable, perhaps a debilitating, draining and *depressing* fight. And depressed people are among the least able to push back, the least able to advocate for themselves. Andrew Solomon writes of patients committing suicide after insurers had them prematurely discharged from hospital. Like the employee who was told he couldn't visit his family in Newfoundland, depressives are very likely to quit their jobs and go away.

I was different. I had no plans to fade away.

CHAPTER 21

Berries

The book tour *was* therapeutic. The public was receptive, the reviews were mostly nice and the interviewers were benign. I stopped feeling like a total loser. The tour lifted my mood considerably, but once back in Toronto with all the reminders of my workplace situation, I retreated into my black hole. Dr. Menchions started me on a new antidepressant, Celexa, while remaining on a full dose of the old one, Cipralex.

Mornings were hardest. Study after study has shown that most suicides occur between 7 A.M. and 4 P.M., and now I can understand why. I would awaken at 3 A.M., and realize that I had another entire endless day to endure. By late afternoon, my misery would ease and by evening, I usually felt somewhat better, knowing the day was ending and I could finally drug myself into oblivion. At bedtime, I would tuck an Ativan under my tongue. As the tranquilizer dissolved into sweet slurry, I would feel my limbs melt and my jaw relax and then I'd slip into a chemical sleep.

In the morning, I was often too drugged and despondent to get out of bed. The boys would leave for school without seeing me. I felt worthless. What kind of parent, a parent who isn't even working, fails to get up and make breakfast for her kids? I couldn't do my job as a journalist. I couldn't write my books. And now I couldn't even fulfill the minimum requirements of a decent mother.

Once I no longer had a friendly escort picking me up and taking me to events, I came scarily close to missing at least two speaking engagements. And when I did make the occasional speech, I almost always ended up in tears. I can't imagine what the organizers thought.

As usual, I wept at my weekly appointment with Dr. Menchions. Unlike me, he had noted how much time was passing. He suggested that distancing myself from my employer might help me recover faster.

"This is not a cost-less thing for you," he warned. "No doubt the circumstances of your workplace are prolonging your depression. You are by nature highly competitive. It's propelled you to tremendous success. But at some point, it's worth walking away from the *Globe*. Don't let the bloodlust [for winning] crowd out everything."

My doctor was providing classic psychiatric advice: avoid strife, retreat, take shelter. But in my case this reasonable approach didn't work. I was fighting for my most basic rights as a journalist and as a human being—the right to speak, the right to be ill. It would be *more* damaging for someone like me to walk away in defeat. If I capitulated, I feared I would end up broken in spirit. I might never recover.

I began spending even more time in stores. It seemed a sociable but safe way to be around other people without the obligation of real intimacy. Unfortunately, despite my pay stoppage, I continued my career as a reckless shopaholic. It had started with the purchase of those shoes in Scottsdale and escalated to that slinky cocktail dress, which had cost a breathtaking seven hundred and fifty dollars. Price, however, had nothing to do with my new pastime. I was happy in dollar stores, too. When I had ten minutes available before a doctor's appointment, I bought crystal candlesticks. In the spare five minutes before meeting friends at the theater, I dashed into Payless Shoes and bought a cheap pair of strappy black sandals. On my way to the Royal Ontario Museum, I ducked into Talbots and emerged with a pair of black trousers to add to my collection of seventeen other pairs of black trousers. I walked past a neighborhood shoe store and spied some floral sling-backs in the window. I immediately bought a pair for sixty-eight dollars, even though I would never wear such flimsy flats. At another store, on my way into the subway, I paused long enough to buy two pairs of expensive orthopedic shoes, knowing I would never wear them, either.

I found myself inside a gourmet shop and bought costly vintage sherry vinegar. I wandered into a bookstore and bought four books, none of which I particularly wanted to read. At an airport, a place I normally never shop because prices are so inflated, I snapped up not one but two wool sweaters. After brunch one Saturday with friends, we popped into an antique store on a whim. They bought nothing; I came out with two framed botanical prints.

When Gigi came to Toronto for one of my arbitrations, we dropped by a home appliance store. I watched someone demonstrate an iron that pneumatically sprang up whenever you set it down. I don't even iron and I can't remember why a pop-up iron was supposed to be helpful, but I was all ready to buy one. I only desisted when my sister intervened, firmly, three times.

Another day I came perilously close to buying a mink coat. I happened to pass a fur salon in a downtown department store and felt myself drawn in. I caressed the silky pelts—pearly white, champagne, chocolate brown, gleaming black. I tried on one of the coats. It fell to my ankles and suddenly

I felt strong, rich and confident. In a trance, in front of a triple mirror, I mimed a supermodel's movements. I flipped up the collar, dug my hands in the satiny pockets and shrugged nonchalantly. The coat cost—only $7,000! Regularly $16,999!

A salesman glided over. "We can shorten it for free," he murmured. "We'll monogram it with your name. We'll store it for free, too."

He moved in for the kill. "You look very beautiful in it."

Somehow, I made it home mink-free. Norman listened in wonder and sighed. Then he asked, "Are you nuts?" I didn't deign to answer his question. Deep inside I knew that, yes, I *was* nuts.

It was possible to shop even without entering a store. Inside a subway station, I bought Sam a Toronto Maple Leafs hockey team T-shirt. I spoke at a charity fundraiser and bought an espresso machine at the silent auction table (even though we already had a decent espresso machine at home). I took a shortcut through an underground mall and signed up for a $1,900 refinishing of my dining-room table. Even when I stayed home, merchandise found me. A telemarketer offered me a seven-day subscription to the *Toronto Star* for the price of the Saturday and Sunday papers alone. Although I was still allergic to newspapers, I found myself readying my credit card.

"Okay," I said.

The telemarketer hadn't finished his spiel.

"Yes, I'll take it," I said.

"You'll take it?" he asked, sounding surprised.

"Yes." And I read him my Visa card number.

One hundred and fifty years ago, Flaubert understood the emotional tug of shopping. In *Madame Bovary*, his bored heroine is trapped in a loveless marriage to a dull, provincial doctor and frantically tries to shop her way to happiness—with tragic consequences. Each time *I* bought something, even a stupid hockey T-shirt, I felt inexplicably happy.

"Why is shopping therapeutic?" I asked my psychiatrist.

"Because dopamine is released in the brain."

Shopping activates the brain's reward center, releasing a gush of dopamine, the same happy chemical triggered by gambling, drug use and other addictive behaviors. You actually have to purchase something, by the way. British scientists found that window-shopping does nothing for dopamine release. They discovered a marked difference in brain patterns between shoppers who are just browsing and shoppers who are about to buy. (Just like I actually had to *go* somewhere; a stay-at-home vacation just didn't cut it for me.)

But *why* did shopping release dopamine? Dr. Menchions wasn't sure.

Allow me to share my own theory with you: evolution. Just as depression results from a sustained flood of fight-or-flight cortisol, retail therapy might likewise be rooted in our primitive juices. After all, we are descendants of successful shopaholics, the ones who enjoyed gathering roots and berries so much that they gathered more than they actually needed. They might not have *consciously* accumulated a surplus. They merely had the type of brain that released a squirt of dopamine when they found another berry patch, and another, and whoa! Another! Those gatherers whose brains didn't release the pleasure hormone found just enough for dinner—and then quite reasonably went back to the cave for a nap. The next day if a hurricane destroyed all remaining berries, they starved. Meanwhile, the shopaholics of the Neolithic era would have survived another day—and had another chance to pass down their genes to us.

Far-fetched? Certainly, the atavistic instinct of the hunter is alive and well today. In *The Omnivore's Dilemma*, Michael Pollan writes about the "ecstasy of the kill" that reaches back to hunter-gatherer economies. After shooting a wild boar in Sonoma, California, he felt a "powerful upwelling of pride" and was "slightly embarrassed to admit" that he felt "absolutely terrific—unambiguously *happy*." He asks, "So how is it we can still go back to being Paleolithic? Because our identity as hunters is literally prehistoric—is in fact inscribed by evolution in the architecture of our bodies and brains."

If hunting remains such a thrill, gathering might similarly be inscribed in the architecture of our brains. As one who has no primal urge to dash through the jungle with a high-powered rifle to find a pot roast, I posit that gathering—shoes, for instance—can be as exciting as hunting (and a lot tidier, too).

With the Internet, gathering is now effortless. I'd be sitting at my computer, minding my own business, when three emails would land in my inbox. *Bling! Bling! Bling!* Did someone design that Pavlovian bell to sound exactly like the nineties word for glitzy stuff? It's hard to concentrate when unsolicited email messages, many with enticing graphics and eye-catching animation, inform me of a 70-percent-off sale on pots and pans at Paderno.com; a time-limited, $10 gift certificate from L.L.Bean.com; a sleek coffee table from CrateandBarrel.com; free delivery on Amazon book orders *today only!*; a designer-dress sale in a stranger's home a five-minute drive away; and a set of animated reindeer lawn ornaments from Walmart. com. I bought the frying pans and books. I went to the stranger's home and picked out a pair of tailored trousers, a pretty aqua top and a floor-length black lace gown by Simon Chang. I wanted to order the illuminated reindeer too, but Norman put his foot down.

One of the most dangerous places to visit when you're depressed is a La-Z-Boy store. Just before one of my arbitrations, Gigi suggested we drop by an outlet, you know, "just to look." I emerged from the furniture store an hour later, several thousand dollars poorer. Apparently, according to Gigi, I shouldn't buy a pop-up iron, but, hey! No problem with a huge yellow recliner *and* a chunky green sofa.

Six weeks flew by, and then the movers were at the door. "Where do you want the recliner?" one of them asked. That was a good question. I led him into the kitchen and showed him a small spot in front of the fireplace. He looked dubious. "And the sofa?"

Another good question. I had no space in my living room, which already accommodated two full-sized sofas, a couple of wing chairs, an overstuffed armchair with matching ottoman, a Chinese armoire, two antique Chinese bookcases, a Qing dynasty *chaise longue* and two coffee tables—not to mention my desk, filing cabinets and office chair. Oh, yes! And a piano. I pointed to a spot beside the piano. It would block pedestrian access to the living room, but it was a spot.

Sam came home from school and surveyed the disaster. "Why do you keep shopping?" he asked, annoyed. "You shouldn't buy anything again without Colleen there to approve." I burst into tears. It was true. Not only was I a shopaholic, I also had appalling decorating taste.

Sam took one look at my wet face and escaped to shoot hoops in the driveway with two of his classmates. I was sitting glumly in the living room on my chunky, green La-Z-Boy sofa when Sam's two friends, Daryl and Sean, came inside.

"What a nice sofa!" exclaimed Daryl.

"We really like your sofa!" Sean chimed in.

Absurdly, I began to smile. Sam crept in behind them. He led his friends into the kitchen to show them the bulky yellow recliner. I followed.

"It's too big," I wailed.

"No," said Sean firmly. "It's really nice."

"Yeah," said Daryl, nodding vigorously.

"Really?" I asked eagerly. And at the time my reporter's skepticism was so completely sublimated that I believed them.

When I wasn't weeping, I was often angry. After my family and I had come under attack in Quebec, I had asked for support from the Canadian

Journalists for Free Expression. No one responded. Later, when my sick pay had been stopped and I'd been silenced, I approached PEN Canada, an organization dedicated to helping writers in distress, and they had turned me down, saying my case seemed to be a "labor-management dispute." The day I got the latest rebuff, I lost it. I yelled at Sam to stop watching television. I ordered him to start practising cello. I hollered at Ben for no reason at all. Sam sulked, but Ben tried to understand. He gave me a hug and said, "It's good you're going to Shanghai tomorrow."

Yes, I was leaving again. Like an addict, I was seeking another dose of the geographic cure. After the prime minister of Canada criticized me, word of my troubles had spread over the Internet to China. My friend Julie phoned from Shanghai. "Jan, you must come here. Come for a month, two months, however long you can." I leapt at the chance and booked a ticket with my air miles. I planned to be gone for at least a month.

On that last evening home with the boys, I robotically cooked dinner. We ate in silence, everyone still seething from my latest outburst. Then I hurried off to a rehearsal with my flute group. I stared at the tracks in the subway station. In all this time I had had no support from any media or journalism organization. It seemed that no one would speak up in my defence. The rebuff from the writers' society was the last straw. I felt abandoned and betrayed. I hadn't received my sick pay in months. My book on maids was in jeopardy over the demand that I pay for the used notes. And now my boys were angry with me.

There must have been other people waiting on the subway platform, but I didn't see them. I looked down and saw the silver tracks, so seductively shiny, so mesmerizing and smooth. They didn't look like they could hurt. I could end it all quickly. I visualized myself stepping in front of a train. There would be no blood, no gore, no screams—at least, that's how I visualized it. It would be a clean, sterile, tidy, quiet end.

As the train roared into the station, I stood rooted to the spot. Part of me felt numb. The other part felt shocked: for the first time in my life I had contemplated killing myself.

Nearly 2 percent of deaths worldwide are suicides, according to the World Health Organization. That makes suicide more lethal than murder *and* war put together. In the past half-century, for reasons no one quite understands, the suicide rate has surged by 60 percent worldwide. From 1999 to 2004, the latest year studied, the U.S. Centers for Disease Control and Prevention found that the mid-life suicide rate among forty-five to fifty-four year olds increased by nearly 20 percent. In both developed and developing countries, suicide is now the second major killer (after tuberculosis) of women between the ages of fifteen and forty-four. For men, it is the fourth leading cause of death (after traffic accidents, tuberculosis and violence.)

As I've mentioned before, men are four times as likely to kill themselves. But there are national exceptions that no one seems able to convincingly explain. China, for instance, has a higher rate of female suicides (even though it has lower rates of postpartum depression than other countries). In 1990, more than 180,000 Chinese women committed suicide, accounting for *more than half* the world's female suicides. Many of these Chinese women lived in rural areas and killed themselves by drinking readily available pesticide.

Suicides everywhere are little understood, but they do have a seasonal pattern, according to Kay Redfield Jamison in her book, *Night Falls Fast: Understanding Suicide*. April is indeed the cruelest month. Records ranging from fifteenth-century England to twentieth-century America show there is a dramatic spike in suicides each spring. Contrary to expectation, she notes, the suicide rate plummets during the darkest months of winter. Can the seasonal variation be related in some way to the dread depressives feel each morning, compared with a relative improvement in mood as the skies darken each afternoon? Can a darkened environment soothe a depressed person, the way sad music is a balm?

Suicide often occurs during the acute phase of depression, although there is no correlation between suicide and the severity of a depression. Paradoxically, the riskiest time for patients is at the beginning of treatment, when they first start taking antidepressants. The mood remains gloomy, but suddenly the patient has enough energy to carry out a plan.

One in five people suffering from major depression, particularly those experiencing their first episode, will attempt suicide. Ten to 15 percent of depressed patients eventually die by suicide. Jamison notes that it is the second leading cause of death among college students and third among young adults between the ages of nineteen and twenty-four. Scientists, composers and business executives are five times more likely to kill themselves than the ordinary population. Writers, especially poets, have an even higher rate.

What happened to me on the subway platform was not a suicide attempt. It was only a *thought*. There is a huge gap between thinking about suicide and actually carrying it out. Suicide ideation is common, so common as to be a line on the standard form my psychiatrist had filled out at my first visit. At that time, I had breezily assured Dr. Menchions that I had no intention of killing myself. But now I had glimpsed the dark side. I understood why people don't always go quietly and cleanly, why they don't just swallow a half bottle of vodka and a bunch of pills at bedtime. Suicide is often unplanned. An irresistible opportunity presents itself out of nowhere as a solution to your problems, and you jump.

CHAPTER 22

Flight, Again

On board the flight to Shanghai, the crew passed out a government form that required passengers to disclose whether they suffered from any of the following: psychiatric disorder, STD, leprosy, open pulmonary tuberculosis, AIDS, HIV carrier. I hesitated. And then I figured that if the Chinese authorities were lumping mental illness in with contagious diseases, it was best they didn't know.

I looked forward to seeing Julie. Like so many of my friends, I had met her through my work, four years earlier, when I had written an eleven-part series on Thorncliffe Park, an immigrant neighborhood in Toronto. I had profiled three families there, from Afghanistan, Pakistan and China. Julie and her husband, William, had come to Canada a year earlier from China bringing their entire savings of one hundred thousand dollars. Their plan was simple: Julie would have a baby and William would find a job. They were both thirty-something, fluent in English, confident and ambitious. She had a degree in piano from the Wuhan Conservatory of Music and had owned several Chinese-medicine clinics in Lahore, Pakistan. He had a master's degree in engineering from China, an MBA from Australia and years of managerial experience in manufacturing and international trade.

Julie gave birth to a baby boy, as planned. Six months later, I got a desperate call. Her husband had still not found work and, after two years of keeping up appearances—a good suit for William, a second-hand Toyota RAV4—their money had run out. Over the phone, Julie sobbed so hard I could hardly make out what she was saying. I knew very little then about depression, but I had experienced the postpartum blues. I told her that was probably what she had, and assured her it was both commonplace and treatable. I urged her to see a doctor. Julie listened to me, and was prescribed antidepressants.

Over the next year, Colleen and I would take Julie out for tea, sweets and walks. She slowly recovered. And then William found the perfect job—as a purchasing manager in Shanghai for the biggest auto-parts manufacturer in Canada. The family returned to China with all the perks and status of expatriate employees at a multinational corporation.

"We have a maid and a chauffeur," Julie had enthused over the phone.

"Just come here and relax."

Her driver picked me up at the Shanghai airport and drove me to their luxurious three-bedroom condo in a gated suburban community. I was starving after my flight from Toronto and devoured the snack their live-in maid had prepared for me: a plate of refreshing pomelo and a bowl of piping hot congee, topped with bok choy from the thriving vegetable garden on their twenty-fifth-floor terrace. Sated, I inspected the condo. It was as luxurious as any in Canada, with hardwood floors, stainless-steel appliances and granite bathrooms.

Before I went to sleep, I made the mistake of checking my email. The union rep had left a message. He was the one who had exclaimed (in an email) about the impropriety of playing shinny during a stress leave. I began trembling. That night I had a nightmare. The rep kept asking, "How come you're vacationing in Shanghai?" I woke up drained.

"Don't phone," Julie advised the next morning. "Just email him. Tell him that talking on the phone makes you sicker."

For months now, the union had been pressing me to return to the office. When I wouldn't cave, it began to see me as the problem. It had already washed its hands of my long-term disability claim on the basis that this benefit was outside the collective agreement. And it made clear that it resented the mounting legal expenses, not to mention its own fraying relationship with management.

Julie tried her best to help. Seeing that I was suffering from severe constipation, a side effect of the antidepressants, she took me to the walk-in clinic at Ren Ji, one of Shanghai's best hospitals. The walk-in part was literal: patients walked in and stood in line before a doctor sitting in the middle of the main lobby who listened (along with everyone else in line) to what ailed you. When my turn came, I talked in self-conscious whispers. The journalist in me wondered which public admission was more humiliating: depression or constipation? They seemed about par.

The doctor, a slim woman in a fashionable, cranberry-red down jacket, heard me out and tapped a few keystrokes on her laptop, sending my prescription for laxatives to the pharmacy on the far side of the lobby. Then she turned to the next person in line.

I wasn't finished. "I want those things that you stick in your anus," I whispered as primly as possible. I didn't know the Mandarin word for "suppository," but for some reason I knew the word for "anus". The doctor nodded expressionlessly and typed rapidly, sending a second prescription to the pharmacy.

Alas, she had interpreted "those things that you stick in your anus" as enemas, which I discovered back at Julie's condo. Inside a small white package were a dozen long-stemmed plastic bulbs filled with lavender liquid. I had never used an enema before so I carefully followed the Chinese instructions. My humiliation was complete.

The union rep emailed me with bad news. After requesting my doctor's complete clinical notes, a list of all my medications and a record of all my psychiatric sessions, *and* after six months of delay, the Manulife intervention specialist had formally abstained from ruling on my short-term claim. Her inaction left in place the *Globe's* assertion that I wasn't sick, which meant my employer would not have to pay me sick pay.

By now I was supposed to be collecting long-term disability. But as short-term disability was the precondition for long-term disability, Manulife would not have to pay a dime either. So much for those promised, tax-free monthly checks. I began to weep.

"You must fight them," Julie said firmly.

It's hard to fight an insurance giant, even if you're Barack Obama's mother. When she was dying at age fifty-three, she fought her insurance company, trying in vain to prove her cancer had not been a pre-existing condition. In my case, I had zero leverage. I paid 100 percent of the premiums, but my employer chose the insurance company. This being the case, only my employer had the clout to fight for my claim. Instead my employer was fighting *me*.

To distract me, Julie took me shopping. At Shanghai's newest malls, the dopamine flowed as I purchased armloads of pashminas and freshwater pearl necklaces for friends back home. I scooped up fleece jackets for Norman and the boys. I bought myself leather boots, extra pairs of prescription glasses and another silver flute. Anticipating the day I would return to work, I ordered custom-made tweed suits and silk dresses from Shanghai's famed tailors. And then I bought a knock-off Samsonite suitcase to lug the loot home.

One day, William had a business meeting in Suzhou, an ancient city on the lower reaches of the Yangtze River, and invited me to tag along so I could see the sights. During the ninety-minute drive, I noticed an intermittent swooshing in my right ear. It sounded a bit like surf. I assumed some water had gotten inside my ear when I showered the night before. I shook my head, but couldn't dislodge whatever it was.

Back in Shanghai that evening, Julie and I watched a DVD, *Elizabeth*, starring Cate Blanchett. I couldn't quite hear the dialogue, but Julie wouldn't let me turn up the volume. She said if it were any louder, it would disturb the maid. I gave up and went to bed. Besides, I was leaving the next day on a side trip to Beijing.

When I called Julie from the airport to thank her for her hospitality, she could hear me fine, but I could barely hear her. On the flight to Beijing, the swooshing sound in my right ear became a low buzz. After the plane landed, I called my friend, Ke, for directions to her home. Like Julie, she could hear me, but I couldn't hear her. Frustrated, I passed my cellphone to the taxi driver, who had no problem getting the directions. When he gave me my phone back, I happened to put it against my other ear.

The cellphone wasn't malfunctioning. I had gone deaf in my right ear. I freaked. How could I work as a reporter if I couldn't hear? How could I play in the band? And then this thought: *Oh, now she's pretending she's deaf, too.*

I arrived at Ke's home on the verge of hysteria. She tried to calm me by suggesting the problem was likely temporary, perhaps caused by cabin pressure during the flight. I thought maybe the mishmash of medications I'd been taking might be to blame. Whatever the problem was, I was already late for a dinner date with Scarlet, my Peking University roommate. I told Ke I'd be back in the evening.

Half an hour later, I was sitting in Scarlet's kitchen while she cooked me some pork-and-cabbage dumplings. When I blurted out that I had suddenly gone deaf in my right ear, she said instantly, "It's because you're tired." That took me by surprise. I hadn't even mentioned what a lousy year it had been. I gave her the super-short summary. Although most of my friends in Canada had been aghast when I told them what had happened, Scarlet wasn't.

"Capitalism, socialism, they're all the same. If leaders have power, they abuse you. You have to ignore them and get on with your life. We've all learned to do that in China."

The next morning, it sounded as though the entire Atlantic Ocean had flowed into my right ear. I now had to turn sideways to hear when someone spoke to me. Ke insisted I get checked out. Right after breakfast she drove me to a private clinic where a cheerful American doctor scrutinized my bag of medications and quickly ruled them out as the cause.

"Your eardrum is intact," she said, peering inside my ear. "There's no wax build-up, no inflammation. It's not mechanical either. That means it's nerve-related. Something is affecting the nerve in your ear. Been to any rock concerts lately?"

"Not in the last thirty years," I said.

She typed a few words into her computer. I looked over her shoulder as a web page flashed up. "Sudden sensorineural hearing loss ... permanent ... catastrophic hearing loss..."

Frightened, I asked what it all meant.

"Sometimes SSHL is caused by the herpes virus, but you have no rash. It could be the result of a blood clot that is blocking the blood vessel. In other words, a minor stroke in the ear. But most of the time, it's idiopathic."

"Idiopathic?"

"That means no one has a clue."

The doctor wrote me a prescription for anti-viral drugs on the off chance it was a herpes-related virus. She also added a massive dose of steroids to reduce swelling. "It's the only Western treatment that has any effect."

She left the room to consult with a Chinese colleague down the hall. When she returned, she wrote a third prescription, for gingko pills. "Apparently there's a traditional Chinese treatment that involves gingko. You really should see a specialist right away." The doctor tried to make me an appointment at the hospital affiliated with the clinic. Unfortunately the specialist was fully booked that day.

I walked out, stunned. *Permanent. Catastrophic.*

Ke urged me to go to the hospital anyway and talk my way in. "You're a journalist," she reminded me. "You can do it."

United Family Hospital was a for-profit facility catering to well-heeled foreigners and China's nouveau-riche capitalist class. The gleaming white, five-storey building was spotless, with automatic sliding glass doors, vases of fresh lilies and copies of *Architectural Digest*.

"We have no more ENT appointments left for today," the receptionist said politely.

I nodded agreeably and said I would wait in case of a cancellation. I sat down on a sleek white sofa in full view of the receptionist. After twenty minutes, I approached her again, smiling sweetly. This time, I stood in front of her desk, and wouldn't budge.

She made a phone call.

"The doctor wants to know what the problem is," she said, covering the mouthpiece.

I told her I had suddenly lost hearing in one ear. She spoke again into the phone.

"The doctor can see you in half an hour."

Sudden sensorineural hearing loss, it turns out, is a recognized health emergency in China. The specialist, a thirty-five-year-old, rosy-cheeked doctor, spoke English but was more comfortable with Mandarin. She clamped some bulky earphones over my ears and handed me a small device, instructing me to push the button whenever I heard something. After ten minutes, she removed the earphones.

"Your left ear is normal. Your right ear is a problem, especially with high-frequency sounds. You are basically deaf." I listened in shock as she rattled off some statistics. SSHL is defined as a hearing loss of at least thirty decibels, half the volume of normal conversation, in three contiguous frequencies. Only two out of three patients ever regain their hearing, sometimes spontaneously. If there is profound hearing loss over the entire spectrum, the prognosis is grim.

My particular hearing loss was profound and spectrum wide.

The doctor said there was hope if patients begin treatment in the first twenty-four hours. After forty-eight hours, the chance of recovery is slim. After seven days, the loss is permanent. With dread I calculated that it had been sixty hours since the swooshing sound began in my ear.

"This is an acute emergency," the doctor said.

I stared at her.

"Most of the time, it's because your inner ear lacks blood," she continued. "In rare cases, it could be a tumor on the nerve, which we'd see through an MRI or a CAT scan. But the most common cause is fatigue and stress."

"I'm depressed," I blurted.

She nodded, as if she heard that all the time. "You have to relax, get decent sleep. It's all related to unhappiness. If your emotions are bad, your blood vessels constrict."

Unhappiness had made me deaf? Was that even possible?

I willed myself not to cry. I had to focus on what the doctor was saying. She guessed that stress was constricting the cochlear artery, restricting blood flow and starving the nerve in my inner ear. She prescribed a intravenous drip of steroids and gingko biloba, manufactured by a Sino-German joint venture and available only in Germany and China. The steroids would reduce inflammation and swelling. The gingko, distilled from the fan-shaped leaves of the Chinese maidenhair tree, would promote circulation and expand my blood vessels.

The doctor said I had to start the two-hour intravenous treatment at once—in the emergency room. I should continue daily treatments for at least ten days, possibly longer. My head spinning, I told her I'd only planned to be in Beijing three more days. I babbled about my return plane tickets to Shanghai and Toronto. I mentioned plans for a weekend in Tianjin. The doctor urged me to cancel everything. In a daze, I followed a nurse down the hall to start my treatment.

"My husband has the same thing," the nurse confided, when she saw how upset I was. "It's so competitive now in Beijing. Lots of high-school students have sudden deafness. Maybe it's the pollution, or maybe the stress. Yours is definitely stress-related."

Within minutes, I was lying on a clean bed, hooked up to an IV bag filled with a bright yellow liquid. Swallowing back tears, I thanked the doctor for staying late on a Friday night to take care of me.

"You must relax," she urged, as she watched me cry.

After the nurse pulled shut the pale green privacy curtains encircling my bed, I no longer fought the tears. They flowed freely down my cheeks and onto my neck, soaking the pillow. I had toughed out sleepless nights, muscle twitches, enemas, too. I had lost my self-esteem, my memory, my salary and my sanity. Now I had lost the hearing in one ear. Sudden deafness was Nature's melodramatic way of grabbing my attention. Stress was not benign.

And that's when I finally decided it was time to quit my newspaper. Lying flat on my back, alone in a foreign hospital, deaf in one ear, with a stainless-steel needle sticking out of my right hand, I suddenly saw matters more realistically. After my first bout of depression, I had returned to the newsroom and seen how dysfunctional it was, how unhappy and anxious my colleagues were. But I had not seen how unhappy and anxious *I* was. Now I understood that I could not return to the newsroom without seriously risking my health, and not just my mental health, but my physical well-being, as well.

My tears fell harder. I wept over my hearing loss. I wept, too, for the loss of what I once thought was the best job in the world. Blindly, I rummaged through my backpack for a tranquilizer and stuck it under my tongue. I had never expected to end my journalism career, severely constipated, drugged on a benzo, hooked to an IV of gingko extract in a hospital in Beijing. As the professor said, I'd had a good run. Now it was over.

CHAPTER 23

Year of the Rat

My friends, Ke and her husband, Ben Mok, came that night to the hospital to fetch me. They were alarmed to find me, weeping, in the emergency room. Ben was a classmate from McGill University who now ran a division of Coca-Cola in China. He and his wife welcomed me to stay with them for the duration of my gingko-steroid treatment.

I phoned home. Norman, upset, urged me to cancel all travel plans. Ben felt as helpless and worried as if I had been in a car accident. Sam, by then fourteen, said, "Mom, just have a good cry. It will make you feel better."

Gigi replied instantly to my email. Like Norman, she told me to heed the doctor and stay in Beijing for treatment. I emailed my friend Talin, the CBC radio producer. She leaped into action, immediately forwarding pages of helpful but alarming research to me.

Sudden sensorineural hearing loss, I learned, is one of the most perplexing mysteries in otolaryngology, the branch of medicine concerned with ear, nose, throat and head-and-neck disorders. Each year, about four thousand people in the United States, mostly between the ages of thirty and sixty, suddenly go deaf, often permanently, usually in one ear, sometimes in both.

I canceled my travel plans. That night in the shower, I could hear water splashing on my left ear, but not on my right. I rubbed my finger over my left ear and listened to the soft swish of skin on skin. I rubbed my right ear. Nothing. Tears ran down my face.

Before I went to sleep, I organized my ever-expanding array of medications. With the addition of all the new prescriptions from Ke's clinic, my senior-citizen pill case could no longer hold everything. I counted: I was now up to twenty-two pills a day. To put that in perspective, the average number of pills for a nursing-home resident is nine. I had tranquilizers; sleeping pills; 225 milligrams of Effexor, comprised of one small gray gel capsule of 75 milligrams and one large fleshy pink gel capsule of 150 milligrams; potions and pills for constipation. For deafness, my latest affliction, I had: bitter-tasting, ox-blood red gingko pills; shiny red Vitamin B12 pills that turned my urine electric yellow; and round, white steroid pills, handfuls of which I had to gobble several times a day. It was so complicated I drew up a chart to show what time I had to take which meds.

That Saturday and Sunday, I had intravenous treatment. On Monday morning, Dr. Lin Zhonghui, the hospital's ear, nose and throat specialist, gave me the bad news. On average, only 20 percent of patients with my type of wide-spectrum hearing loss ever recovered. The good news was his success rate was way above average. The previous year he had treated twenty patients like me and fully 80 percent recovered.

"I think your deafness is related to your depression," said Dr Lin. He added that Beijing had numerous cases of sudden sensorineural hearing loss due to widespread stress during China's economic boom. He advised me to avoid loud environments and gave me latex earplugs to protect my right ear from excessive noise. "No tea, coffee or alcohol. No caffeine except for green tea. You must relax. That is critical."

I simplified my life. I cancelled eight appointments with friends. I quit shopping at noisy malls. Each morning, I had a quiet breakfast with Ben and Ke and their two young boys. Then I splurged on a taxi to the hospital. In a sunny private room with clean linen and a spotless en suite bathroom, I underwent an IV treatment that often lasted two or three hours. It was so relaxing I often managed a nap. After one week, my hands became scarred with puncture marks and purple-yellow bruises. I began to sympathize with drug addicts, especially when the nurses treating me had trouble finding fresh veins.

After each IV session, I would walk two blocks to my favorite Sichuan restaurant for a solitary lunch. I would order all the spicy dishes no one seemed able to make correctly outside China: diced chili chicken with crunchy peanuts; *ma po* tofu with tongue-numbing, crushed flower-peppercorns; unctuous return-to-the-wok, sliced pork belly; shredded-turnip puffs; *dan dan* noodles with fiery minced pork and preserved vegetables; slivered *yuxiang* pork with pickled red chilies, tree-ear fungus and fresh bamboo shoots; and hot and sour soup properly spiked with finely ground white pepper. Every day I took the abundant leftovers home to supplement dinner with the Mok family.

I had left most of my antidepressants back in Shanghai and soon ran out of Effexor and sleeping pills. I was surprised, but I guess I shouldn't have been, that the same brands were readily available in China. Dr. Lin prescribed more Effexor and Imovane. He wanted to ensure I got plenty of sleep, especially the kind that encourages dreams. "REM sleep is good. It promotes circulation."

One night, after everyone had retired and the house was quiet, I lay in bed listening to the wall clock ticking above my head. I buried my good ear in the pillow. Elated, I found I could now hear a faint tick!

Then I woke up. It had all been a dream.

I discovered I could sometimes direct my dreams. In one, I was promoted to editor-in-chief! My first executive move: free food for everyone in the company cafeteria. My second move: firing the vice-president of human resources. Next I demoted my foes. I reassigned the editor-in-chief to a night-shift, copy-editing slot. I sent his nasty deputy to a remedial writing course (something management sometimes did to humiliate veteran reporters.)

Food for the masses, oblivion for the ruling class—my dream was so delicious, I didn't want to wake up! When I finally did, my first thought each morning was: will I regain my hearing? As a kid, I had attended Sunday school because I liked singing in the choir. When I was old enough to understand the sermons, I decided I was a heathen. Yet whenever I was out of options, like the time Mom underwent quadruple bypass heart surgery, I would sheepishly utter a prayer. God had never held my lack of faith against me. Now, on the fifth day of my deafness, I prayed To Whom It May Concern.

Please, heal my right ear.

Two days later, I was in the shower washing my hair when I suddenly heard the sound of water splashing on my right ear. I snapped my fingers. I could hear something! I rubbed my ear. I could hear skin against skin! My heart leapt. I wasn't dreaming. I immediately phoned Norman to tell him my hearing might be returning. "Say something," I ordered, and then I switched the receiver to my bad ear. To my dismay I could hear nothing. I put the receiver back on my good ear. Suddenly I heard a high-pitched whine. Then nothing.

"Hello? Hello?" I shouted frantically.

Norman called back. "Sorry," he said, "the line went dead on my end."

My husband's voice has always been the same frequency as white noise. That day, while I could not hear him, I began to hear crunchy, metallic sounds when Ke's ten-year-old son practised piano. A few days later, the buzzing in my right ear subsided. Ordinary speech began sounding like low-pitched, plastic clicks.

Excited, Dr. Lin scheduled another audio test. I clamped on the heavy earphones and held my breath. I could hear the beeps! I kept squeezing the gizmo in my hand. When it was over, the doctor beamed. "Congratulations. Your low tones are improved by 20 percent. Your high frequencies are up by 50 percent." He drew a graph and marked my progress in red ink. The line curved sharply up. With a big smile, he prescribed four more days of treatment and told me he fully expected I would continue to improve.

To celebrate, I decided to break the no-caffeine and no-noise rules. I headed for the most expensive mall in Beijing and ordered a cappuccino and two madeleines—Roquefort and chestnut. Sitting on a hot-pink café chair in Fauchon, a replica of the mother store Ben and I had visited at Place de la Madeleine, I savored my first cup of coffee in two weeks. I pulled out my foam earplug and listened to the click-clack of high-heels walking by. Nothing had ever sounded as sweet.

I couldn't believe my luck. True, I had gone deaf in one ear. But I had had the great good fortune to go deaf in Beijing where I had a friend kind enough to take me to her clinic, where the American doctor recognized an emergency. In Beijing, I had been able to talk my way into a hospital, where the Chinese specialists knew all about sudden sensorineural hearing loss and offered a unique gingko-and-steroid treatment. In Toronto, I would have had to wait weeks, if not months, to see someone. And by then, it would have been too late. For the first time in months, I felt blessed.

As Dr. Lin predicted, my hearing improved steadily. Every day, the white noise in my ear receded and I could hear more and more sounds around me. I no longer felt the need to wear a protective earplug. On February 4, I went for my last evaluation with Dr. Lin. It was the eve of the Lunar New Year and he was leaving the next day to spend the holiday with his elderly parents in Shandong province. As he clamped the heavy earphones on my head, I closed my eyes to concentrate. Suddenly I could hear so many sounds—beeps, low buzzing, shrill rings, all of them beautiful. And then I heard him say the best sounds of all.

"Congratulations! You've made a full recovery." He grinned. The nurse beamed. I wanted to hug them tight. But I was in China, where even a handshake can be considered barbarically physical. Instead, I smiled—no teeth showing—and nodded respectfully.

"It's kind of unbelievable," the doctor said, looking proud and happy. "Almost all my patients get better." He prescribed four more days of intravenous treatment and told me to continue taking vitamin B12 for another month to repair possible nerve damage.

"And try to relax," he said.

"If it happens again, fly back to Beijing," said the nurse, with a smile.

That afternoon, I felt drawn to Yonghegong, a seventeenth-century Buddhist lamasery a few miles north of Tiananmen Square. It means

"Palace of Peace and Harmony," and I felt at peace at last. I had recovered my hearing. And I had made up my mind to leave the *Globe*. Lionel Tiger calls places of worship "serotonin factories." The anthropologist contends that our brains invented religion to knit us together into communities to ensure our survival. As I've said, I'm not religious. When I first came to Beijing at the age of nineteen, I was an ardent Maoist. Nowadays, I'm just another boring atheist. Yet somehow I felt a powerful impulse to give thanks. After all, I'd prayed, and two days later, my hearing returned. Perhaps there was a God, after all.

At Yonghegong, I wandered through a maze of pavilions. Originally built in 1694 for court eunuchs, it became the residence of the future Yongzheng emperor and later a lamasery for Buddhist monks from Mongolia and Tibet. On the eve of the Lunar New Year, it was crowded with worshipers. The air was thick with incense and so cold I could see my breath. Chinese women in high-heeled boots and puffy quilted coats knelt before gilded icons, whose altars were piled high with offerings of kiwi, Fuji apples, sweet biscuits, mandarin oranges individually wrapped in glassine bags, large canisters of vegetable oil for the flickering lamps and green glass bottles of Er Guo Tou, the local eau-de-vie.

Yonghegong is one of Beijing's more spectacular temples, with high vermilion walls and a sea of golden-tiled roofs. Walking through a narrow corridor, I chanced upon the Hall of Medicine. A huge gilded Buddha with painted indigo hair and elongated kohl-rimmed eyes presided in the lotus position. Suddenly it occurred to me that *this* was the place to give thanks. As renowned herbalists, Tibetan Buddhists have a repertoire of two thousand different plants. Perhaps they were among the discoverers of the healing properties of gingko.

I knelt down on a pillow before the altar and clasped my frozen fingertips. I gazed up at the Buddha of Medicine, murmuring words of gratitude. Around me I heard the loveliest sounds: the quiet footsteps of the devout, the dry swish of a straw broom over the stone floor, the icy wind whistling outside. I vowed that noise would never again irritate me. Just then a monk bounded past, whipping a cellphone from the folds of his magenta robes.

"*Wei, wei!*" (Hello, hello!), he shouted into it.

Normally, I would have glared at him. Now I smiled serenely.

Another monk, in a coarsely woven, padded brown robe, cinched at the waist with a red sash, shooed me out. "We're off-duty now. It's closing time."

I smiled again. I could hear him loud and clear.

Just before I left Beijing, I went to see Lu Yi. In 1973, when we were both students at Peking University, we had had a brief, life-changing encounter. Mainly *I* changed *her* life—for the worse. We didn't know one another, but she knew I was from Canada and had stopped me on the campus to ask my help in getting to the United States. Naively—and thoughtlessly—I told my teacher. Shortly thereafter, I returned to Canada.

More than two decades later, I was ending my posting as the *Globe's* China correspondent when my roommate, Scarlet, told me Lu Yi had been expelled. Appalled and ashamed, I wanted to make amends, but no one knew where she had ended up. I didn't think I could find her. And to be honest, I was afraid to find her.

For years, Lu Yi's fate haunted me. Then my publisher commissioned another book on the eve of the 2008 Beijing Olympics. It was finally time to search for the woman I had wronged. In the summer of 2006, one month before the Dawson College shooting, I went to Beijing to find Lu Yi. Thirty-three years had elapsed since our encounter and I didn't even know the Chinese characters for her name. But I deployed every journalistic resource available and ran down every contact. I eventually found her. And then I decided that her story was more important than anything I could write about the Olympics.

That was the book I wrote in the depths of my depression. In fact, it was therapeutic to write about Lu Yi, my search for redemption and her generous forgiveness. Writing *Beijing Confidential* helped me recover sufficiently to return, albeit shakily and briefly, to the newsroom before my complete breakdown. Lu Yi was the main reason I had come to Beijing on this trip; I wanted to present her with a copy of the new book.

"I don't blame you," she said, holding my hand as we sat side by side, drinking green tea in her living room on the campus of Peking University. "You didn't understand what you were doing. I don't hate you. In fact, I admire you. You tried so hard to find me. You weren't afraid to say you were wrong and to admit what you did."

As her husband, a retired professor, refilled our cups, I told them about what had happened to me at work. They said it reminded them of the Cultural Revolution. But when I mentioned my sick pay stoppage, they were shocked. "Even the Communist Party never did that," Lu Yi's husband said.

Yes, yes, I know my sick pay stoppage isn't a crime on a par with genocide. But depression is never about perspective. You can have a full refrigerator and gas in your tank. You can be on your honeymoon with the most wonderful partner in the world. Like William Styron, you can win an international prize and receive a big fat check—and none of this will mitigate your depression. It is what it is.

My Chinese friends seemed to understand. "You became a scapegoat," Lu Yi said, nodding.

We had reservations that evening at a nearby restaurant. Given how I'd ratted her out when I was young, it seemed sardonically appropriate to be celebrating the Year of the Rat. Of course, in China the rat doesn't have the Western connotation of snitching. In the Chinese zodiac, the rat is auspicious: it symbolizes survival and determination.

PART V

HAPPINESS

CHAPTER 24

The Art of War

I returned to Toronto knowing I had to leave my job. Still, I wavered every day. To save my mental and physical health, I had to quit the *Globe*. To save my mental and physical health, however, I could not slink away in defeat.

Dr. Menchions finally understood. "If you were less tenacious, it would probably be better to just walk away. But for you to walk away is to leave a piece of yourself behind."

Paradoxically, "winning" would not constitute a victory. What kind of win is it when you lose what you love? Indeed, I initially defined victory in the only terms a corporation understood: money. Gradually I began to consider what *I* meant by victory: freedom of speech and an acknowledgment that I was truthful when I said I was sick.

Everyone assumed I would return to the paper as soon as I recovered. Only my psychiatrist and my family knew otherwise. Meanwhile I remained severely depressed. I hadn't been paid in a year. A string of arbitrations loomed. And I'd been ordered back to work, yet again, after Manulife's consulting psychiatrist had viewed the Garda videos and said I looked "vivacious."

As cortisol inundated my system, I began having, in the jargon of psychiatry, lots of "suicide ideation." People who actually commit suicide often obsess about it for days. They visualize each step. They stare out the farmhouse window at the barn and see the sturdy rafters. They know exactly how they will knot the rope. But they often can't think beyond the act itself.

I wasn't like that. After my moment on the subway platform, some morbid attraction kept drawing me to the overpass near my house. But whenever I stared at the four-lane road below, I visualized the aftermath. I thought that unless I did a perfect swan dive and landed on my head, a jump wouldn't be fatal. At rush hour, of course, I could reliably depend on an SUV running me over. Then I imagined the impact on my loved ones, the trauma for the SUV driver and the mess for the police and ambulance crew. The ability to picture all this meant I was not that far gone. People who actually commit suicide can't envision the consequences. In *Mrs. Dalloway*, Septimus leapt out a window without anticipating that his wife might find him impaled on the iron fence below.

"Promise me," Talin said one day as we were sitting in my living room having tea. "Promise me you're not going to kill yourself."

I couldn't speak. My eyes filled with tears. I nodded.

One day on the overpass, I suddenly felt some of my old energy flowing back. Had the antidepressants finally kicked in? Was the talk therapy with Dr. Menchions working? Had the depression run its natural course? Had my decision to quit the *Globe* improved my mental state? Perhaps all of these elements helped nudge me onto the trajectory to recovery. I'm not sure. Just as every depression is unique to the individual, every recovery, every emergence, every transition to normalcy is different. Some people get better fast, dramatically, overnight. My recovery began with this surge of energy, but it would not be a smooth path upward towards the light. It would be bumpy and there would be setbacks.

All I know is this: at that moment, standing on the overpass over the busy road, I had ruminated about my situation for the umpteenth time and something snapped. I would not kill myself. Instead, I walked back home and instructed my lawyer to sue Manulife. Then I phoned my literary agent. I told him that although I remained depressed and could not yet write and had no idea when I might be able to write again, I planned to produce a book about my experience with mental illness.

But first I had to recover. I showed my Chinese medical file on sudden sensorineural hearing loss to Dr. Au, who sent me to specialists at St. Michael's Hospital in Toronto. They confirmed my right ear had made a full recovery and were intrigued to hear of the gingko treatment. I asked if there was any validity to the link between hearing loss and depression.

"We do think it's sometimes related to depression and stress," the otolaryngologist-in-chief said. "You were very lucky. You were in the right place at the right time."

The organizers of a book festival in Sydney, Australia, invited me to speak about *Beijing Confidential*. It would be another book tour, another dose of the geographic cure. My Australian publisher arranged several interviews to publicize the book. Everything went swimmingly until a journalist down under surprised me with a question about my absence from the pages of the *Globe*.

"I can't talk about it or I'll be fired," I blurted.

Naturally, she quoted me. I was distraught. I had just broken management's directive banning me from even talking about *why* I couldn't talk. (Indeed, the *Globe*'s lawyers later used that against me at one mediation hearing.)

When the interview was published on the second day of the festival, I couldn't stop crying. For more than a year, I had tried so hard to obey the order, and now I had screwed up.

Shona Martyn, my Australian publisher and a former journalist herself, was kindness incarnate. Normally, publishers take authors out for one bang-up meal per visit. Shona and her staff took me out *every* day. They never let me eat alone. They took me sightseeing and pointed out actor Russell Crowe's waterfront condo. On Sunday, they insisted they had nothing better to do than invite me to brunch, followed by a hike along Bondi Beach. When I mentioned that I hoped to climb the Sydney Harbour Bridge, the publicist surprised me by taking me there and paying for the $198 ticket. She looked the other way while I filled out the pre-climb questionnaire. Like the Chinese health form on the airplane to Shanghai, this one also asked about psychiatric problems (but not leprosy).

My climbing group was small, just four others—a young Brazilian woman, a honeymooning couple from Japan and an Irish doctor who looked like he ran marathons. We watched a safety video first and then donned knit caps, gloves, fleece jackets and khaki jumpsuits. The jumpsuit had a built-in safety chain at the waist that hooked onto a steel cable strung along the entire length of the bridge. I could have circumvented the security system by disrobing, but I had no suicide ideation that involved leaping naked off the world's largest single-span arch bridge.

For three-and-a-half hours, I clambered after our brash Aussie guide. I had to stop occasionally to catch my breath. And whenever I looked down, my knees felt watery and my heart pounded. But for the first time in months I felt alive. I watched the sun set, streaking the sky orange and flamingo, and then indigo. The moon—round and pure as a deep-sea pearl—rose over the Sydney Opera House. Really, it did. At the apex of the bridge's arch, I flung my arms triumphantly in the air. And then I began my descent. By the time my feet were back on solid ground, I knew I was getting better.

I returned home to find that Sam's cello teacher had fired him for failing to practice five lessons in a row. Instead of weeping and blaming myself, I took charge. To Sam's chagrin, I found him an excellent new teacher within forty-eight hours.

Then I got the shocking news that my friend Val Ross had passed away. A few months after we had gone out for that glass of merlot, she had been diagnosed with a brain tumor. Because she hadn't wanted to see anyone (and neither had I), we had only exchanged get-well cards. Her last words to me: "I don't know whether the stress at work caused my brain tumor or my brain tumor caused me to be stressed at work."

Val was fifty-seven. I couldn't believe she was gone. I attended her funeral at the University of Toronto's Massey College, a place she had loved so much as a journalism fellow. By coincidence, I had applied for a similar fellowship at the suggestion of John Fraser, the Master of Massey. Soon after Val's funeral, however, he sent me am email telling me I had been passed over. "The problems seemed a bit too big for the committee … they felt the college and the program would be drawn relentlessly into controversy."

I cried—but not all that much. It was now clear that in a battle between a big newspaper and a lone reporter, there would be no support from any journalism organization. It was the last bit of disillusionment, the last heartbreak. My depression *was* helping me see the world in a clearer way. I was on my way to recovery.

At my next appointment, I asked Dr. Menchions if I could switch from Effexor, my third antidepressant, which I'd been on for six months. I hated the side effects, the dry mouth and dry eyes, and especially the severe constipation. He began stepping down Effexor and started me on 200 milligrams a day of Wellbutrin, an atypical antidepressant that works on multiple neurotransmitters.

My psychiatrist had advised me to visualize a life without the *Globe*. I told him I had reached the point where I was finally able to do that. I considered starting a Mandarin-English private school. I thought about teaching journalism. I dreamed of opening a restaurant. I even contemplated freelancing myself out to rewrite museum signage (which I'd always found numbingly unhelpful).

Psychically, as I moved beyond the workplace, the fight with my newspaper receded in emotional significance. Almost in passing, I mentioned that I had been ordered back to work yet again. Dr. Menchions repeated what he had been saying for months: I was not ready to return. We didn't dwell on it. We went on to other topics.

Afterward, I took the elevator down to the main floor of the bank tower. In the lobby, a well-dressed man caught my eye. We exchanged smiles and nods. A moment later I realized it was the former prime minister of Canada. As a reporter, I'd once followed Jean Chrétien on the campaign trail. He had ignored me then, but we'd later crossed paths at a memorial service for a mutual friend, a Liberal senator. During the reception that followed, to my surprise Chrétien had chuckled and said, "I know who you are. You were a Montreal Maoist." He explained that he had watched a documentary about me on television the night before.

This time in the bank lobby, the former prime minister couldn't place me. Before I could say anything, an aide whispered in his ear. Chrétien nodded and smiled. Then he remarked that my byline seemed to have vanished from the *Globe*.

"I'm depressed," I said. "I can't write."

"That's terrible. What are you doing now?"

I sidestepped the question. Instead I posed one to him. I knew that despite his success as a politician he had suffered setbacks, including losing a leadership race. In the 1980s, his party had gone down to defeat. For a time he'd even quit politics.

"Have you ever been depressed?" I asked.

The former prime minister hesitated. "Sometimes it's very difficult."

"What did you do?"

"You get up in the morning and you fight," Chrétien said. "Every morning, you get up, and it's another day and another fight."

CHAPTER 25

Fired Up

June 4 is imprinted in my memory as the day I covered the Tiananmen Massacre. Nine years later, it was also the day *The Globe and Mail* fired me. Surprisingly I didn't feel another stab of betrayal. Then I understood—I was already one step further on my way to recovery.

The union rep tried to dissuade me from attending the proceedings the following Monday. "It's just a formality," he said. "You don't have to come in. You walk into a meeting. They hand you a letter. That's the end of it."

But after twenty-one years at the *Globe*, I wouldn't dream of missing my own firing. The union rep sighed. "You want to look them in the eye."

I had recently stopped weeping at each psychiatric appointment. I hadn't shed a single tear when I learned I was going to be sacked. But now, as I told my doctor what had happened, my eyes brimmed. "Go ahead and have a good cry," he said. "Usually I tell people to try to understand that it's not personal. But with you, it's personal. And if you understand that, you'll be able to heal."

I broke down in huge wracking sobs. Would other companies reject me because I had suffered from a mental illness?

"Or what if they don't want me because I'm such a pain in the butt?"

"I think they'll want you *because* you are."

Dr. Menchions tried to prepare me for that Monday. "It's an awful thing to go through. It's going to hurt like hell. Nobody ever wants to get fired."

I wondered aloud if it was my fault, if there was anything I should have done differently?

"It's simple," Dr. Menchions said. "You wrote a story. There was a big backlash and your paper didn't back you. All the rest stems from those events."

So it *was* like an Ian McEwan plot after all. I wrote a story and then ... *all the rest stems from those events*. Somehow that calmed me down.

My session was up. My psychiatrist ushered me out the unmarked door into the public hallway. "You're getting better," he said, "but you're still depressed."

Gigi drove in from Montreal to be by my side during my firing. I told her I was upset that I couldn't retrieve my stuff from the office. Thirteen months earlier when I attended the awards dinner in Winnipeg, I had no inkling I would never return to the newsroom. I wanted my things—family photos, shoes, a couple of sweaters, my books, files and notebooks.

"We'll get it over the weekend," my sister said decisively. "They won't expect us to go in."

I began to smile as I pictured the two of us charging through the front doors. Retrieving my belongings suddenly seemed liberating, an act of defiance and derring-do after nearly two years of being unable to do much of anything. Raiding the office would also serve as a dress rehearsal for entering the building on Monday. For a long time I had been too upset to go near the *Globe*.

"You really think we can get the stuff?" I said.

"Sure. Why not?"

Dr. Menchions, who seemed to work ridiculously long hours, had already booked me for a psyche-buttressing appointment at 7:45 A.M. on Saturday, two days before my scheduled firing. Conveniently, his office was a two-minute drive from the *Globe*. And Saturday, it turns out, would be perfect for the raid: the newsroom would be deserted because the newspaper didn't publish the next day, Sunday.

Gigi had obtained permission from Dr. Menchions to attend my session. She wanted to ask how she could help me. "Listening to her is always extremely valuable," Dr. Menchions said. "This depression has slowed her down. She has to get back to a high level of functioning, not just intellectually, but emotionally. She needs that airing out."

My sister told him I'd been exercising poor judgment lately. For example, I had taken Sam to a cello concert the night before his *brevet*, a standardized French-government language exam. She thought I should have kept him at home studying and wondered if she should criticize me.

Dr. Menchions shook his head. "She's got plenty of criticism around her now. The medication hasn't been a silver bullet. I think she's better than she was. She is truly a warrior. She isn't emotionally labile or..."

I felt self-conscious listening to my doctor and sister talk about me. When he called me a "warrior," I felt absurdly pleased. No one had said anything that flattering about me in a long time. But the word "labile" was new to me.

"How do you spell that?" I interrupted.

"L-A-B-I-L-E."

He turned to my sister. "You see? She makes me nervous because she asks about everything she doesn't understand and she writes everything down."

Gigi told him of our plan to clean out my desk. He looked concerned.

"There are emotional pitfalls to going into the *Globe*. If the pass doesn't work or the guard can't let you in, that might feel awful. That will be the exact moment you feel fired."

I told him I really wanted to retrieve my belongings. Then we discussed firing scenarios. I said I hoped to use the meeting to ask questions. "The reporter going out the door," he said with a smile, "shouting questions."

Gigi drove five blocks west across Front Street. At the entrance to the *Globe*'s rooftop parking lot, I pulled out my access pass. Gigi waved it in front of the sensor. The gate wouldn't budge.

"Flip it over," I instructed. Gigi waved the other side of my pass before the sensor.

Nothing happened.

Contrary to my doctor's warning, I didn't feel bad at all. I felt a rush of adrenalin and elation. There would be no more flight. I was finally choosing to fight. I was the aggressor now and, baby, I was gonna have *fun*.

My sister and I noticed that the gate on the down ramp was raised. We exchanged glances. Then Gigi reversed and roared up the wrong side of the ramp. We got out of the car and grabbed several empty duffle bags.

The door to the building, of course, was locked. I waved my dead access pass over the sensor.

"Now what?" said Gigi, looking slightly worried.

"Now we go in the front door."

We walked around to the front of the building and entered the lobby. We still had to get through a set of locked doors to the building's interior. A security guard was sitting behind the reception desk. Just for show, I waved my useless pass in front of the sensor. Then I glanced over at the guard.

I didn't recognize him, which was good. It meant he wouldn't recognize me, either.

"Excuse me," I said. "My pass isn't working. Could you please open the door?"

He began typing into his computer. I held my breath. Had human resources put me on a blacklist? Was he suspicious about why we were carrying empty duffel bags? Suddenly, the doors clicked open. I smiled and waved my thanks.

I was pleased to find my desk intact because at the *Globe* it was common for useful items—books, staplers, scissors, even chairs, *especially* chairs—to disappear when anyone was absent for a few days. But everything was as I had left it, including a four-pack of Bacardi Breezer rum cooler that a clueless publicist had sent thirteen months earlier. While Gigi emptied filing cabinets, I cleaned out my drawers. Like so many people, my workplace seemed to have become my home away from home: I found a toothbrush, dental floss, toothpaste, pantyhose, hay-fever pills, hand cream, emergency makeup and a hairbrush. A package of Tampax was a poignant reminder of how long I had been away. I was now peri-menopausal and had no further need of them.

My sister, ever the cautious accountant, worried someone might catch us in flagrante delicto. She decided to start packing the car. I schlepped the first bag down a flight of steps to the rooftop exit.

Damn! I'd forgotten I also needed an access pass to get out.

More adrenalin flooded my system as I crept down one level to the national department. Surely *someone* was obsessed enough to work on a Saturday morning. *Yes!* In the middle of the vast, empty room, a young man sat staring at a computer screen. I had no idea who he was, which meant he didn't know me, either. I squared my shoulders and walked confidently over.

"Hi," I said. "My pass isn't working and I need to carry a few things out to the rooftop parking lot. Can I borrow your pass?"

"Sure," he said, digging into his pocket.

Forty minutes later, we finished packing. I left behind the Bacardi rum cooler and all *Globe* property except for the small rectangular sign I had once hung on my cubicle divider. It seemed important to take back my name.

After returning the pass to my helpful colleague, we left by the front door, making sure to thank the security guard as we left. Outside, the June sun was shining. I had just taken my first step to liberation. As Gigi drove down the ramp, we started laughing. We were like Susan Sarandon and Geena Davis in *Thelma & Louise*. If only Dad's 1994 champagne Mercedes-Benz was a 1966 blue Thunderbird convertible. Too late, I remembered the security cameras trained on the rooftop parking lot. I regretted not waving goodbye.

On Monday morning, I wore a sleeveless gray knit top, a silky pencil skirt and a solitaire pearl necklace. I thought that if I looked professional, I would not cry. The vice-president of human resources was waiting, along with Sylvia Stead, the deputy editor. They immediately objected to my sister's presence. Gigi, however, smiled pleasantly, nodded at them both, and sat down. The thought occurred to me: *two Wongs do make it right.* Suddenly I saw my sister in a new light. I had never before looked up to her. She was, after all, my *baby* sister. But now I saw how tough and loyal she was, and realized how lucky I was to have her for a sister.

Perhaps flummoxed by Gigi's presence, the vice-president remained standing. So did the deputy editor. I stood, too. It felt like we were in the military. The vice-president handed me my letter of dismissal, which was addressed only to "Ms. Wong." After twenty-one years of employment and a byline, I suddenly had no first name at all. The letter appeared to have been written by a lawyer. It listed six somewhat contradictory reasons for dismissing me: "excessive absenteeism"; "innocent absenteeism"; "insufficient information about the state of my health"; "public activities"; "lack of interest" in coming back to the newsroom; and Manulife's repeated denial of my disability claim.

Still standing, I stated that I was ill, had done nothing wrong and wanted to return to my job as soon as I was well. The vice-president did not respond. Nor did Sylvia, who instead asked whether I still had a company BlackBerry. I didn't—I'd never been issued one—but I returned the second-hand cell phone given to me years earlier. (I hadn't used it when I was sick, and at any rate, the company had cut off cell-phone service in the midst of my relapse.) Then the vice-president asked for my defunct access pass. I handed it over, along with my final expense-account receipts, including the one-night hotel bill in Winnipeg during the National Newspaper Awards.

As I left my workplace for the last time, I didn't feel the least bit suicidal. I didn't even feel sad. I felt only relief. After all, I hadn't cried. I hadn't shouted at them. I hadn't gone postal or fallen apart or lost my dignity. As I left I checked my watch, an old habit from my reporting days. I noted that my firing had taken twenty minutes—about one minute for every year I had worked there.

CHAPTER 26

Hush Money

Ten days after I was fired, the *Globe* launched a twenty-eight-part series on depression, called "Breakdown." It was marvelously written and would go on to win a well-deserved National Newspaper Award. Greenspon, the editor-in-chief, wrote the introduction. "When we began reporting for this project, many of us at *The Globe and Mail* were unaware of the scope of the problem in Canada."

Under the headline, "THE WORKING WOUNDED," the lead story noted that mental illness was costing the Canadian economy $51 billion a year. It said that half a million people missed work each day because of psychiatric problems. "What are employers doing about it?" the article asked. "Not much." Another story in the series declared: "Efforts must also be made to change the workplace culture to reduce the stress that is a common trigger for mental illness. Yet few employers are accommodating, and fewer still reach out to help staffers before they descend into crisis. Employees feel the workplace is where they are least likely to get support."

If I hadn't been fired for suffering from a major depressive episode, I could have contributed a dandy first-person article. This juxtaposition—a newspaper producing an ambitious series about depression in the workplace while dumping a depressed employee—points to a bigger truth. Many corporations are capable of public good, even while failing to follow through privately.

Such contradictory behavior is increasingly common these days, according to the authors of *Snakes in Suits*. Paul Babiak and Richard D. Hare argue that the brisk demand for rattling cages smoothes the ascent of a certain type of person to the corner office. Today corporations recruit executives who exude confidence, strength and calm, which also happen to be typical psychopathic traits. While Hollywood depicts them as cannibals like Hannibal Lecter, most psychopaths in fact aren't interested in eating your liver; they just want the lion's share of money and power.

"Where do these psychopaths go?" they write. "Often, it's to the corporate world." The point isn't that CEOs are psychopaths, but that psychopaths are particularly attracted to management jobs. After all, consider the kind of psychological profile required to commit the deeds routinely described in the business media: pillage a company pension plan, off-load five major divisions without a blink or fire 2,500 people two days before Christmas.

My dismissal had been another turning point. By confiscating my access pass, the *Globe* provided literal closure on my career. As one door closed, another opened—to motherhood. At Gigi's suggestion, I asked my psychiatrist if I could bring my husband and sons to an appointment. One Saturday morning the four of us squeezed onto the leather couch.

My family hadn't been keen on coming. The boys shifted uncomfortably. Norman stared at a spot on the wall over the doctor's left shoulder. No one spoke. Dr. Menchions broke the silence by asking what it was like to be around me. Sam, who had recently turned fifteen, mentioned that two years earlier I couldn't get inside my own front door.

"She was so panicked and crying and shaking," Sam said. "She thought someone was trying to kill her."

"She's not crazy, schizophrenic or demented," my psychiatrist told him. "The stress and anxiety got so big she kind of imploded. She will fully recover."

Norman sighed. "For someone who isn't insane, she requires a lot of humoring."

My doctor laughed out loud. Then he became serious. "Is she less lovable?"

Ben, who was now eighteen, spoke up. "She'll get angry faster or upset faster. Recently, I've been getting kind of fed up." He said he had tried hard to be helpful and understanding, but the situation had gone on for two years.

"So this thing has a shelf life?" Dr. Menchions asked.

"Right," said Ben. "I'm tired of dealing with it."

My psychiatrist nodded. Then he asked Norman if he had anything else to say. My husband sighed again. "She's gotten harder to live with. I just try to be as accommodating as possible. I do what she wants to do or wants done."

I cringed. Hearing my family speak frankly, I realized how awful it had been for them and how tired they were of it all. Dr. Menchions kept nodding as if he'd heard the same comments from other families many times before. He told the boys that I was not a depressed person by nature. Circumstances had pushed me into depression.

"Maybe that's the reason to be less accommodating," Ben said. "By enabling her to wallow in it, we're making it worse."

"You're not enabling her because she'd be that way anyway," the doctor said. "She doesn't need to be coddled. She's not weak or broken. She's depressed."

"Now and then she'll sit us down, talk at us for a while, look for some response," said Ben. "It's clear she's looking for us to agree with her. She leans on us for an answer."

"You do pretty well," Dr. Menchions reassured him. "She's looking for emotional support. She doesn't know how to ask. She only knows how to grill people. Just go over and hug her."

"That's what I do," Sam said.

Our time was up. As my psychiatrist ushered us out, he promised my family that my illness was temporary and I would eventually come out of it. "In the meantime, it's good to not go down with the ship," he said. "Four lives are involved."

The company had fired me three weeks before an arbitration hearing over my sick pay. It was the one for which I had waited a whole year. Now that I'd been terminated, the union piled on more grievances over the gag order, the letters of reprimand and now, of course, wrongful dismissal. Everything was coming to a head. The union was furious that I would not fade away. The company was even angrier. With six more mediations and arbitrations looming, I dreaded the strife. My sister came to the rescue with another dose of the geographic cure.

Normally, I shun bus tours. But Gigi pointed out that this one would take us to a dozen stately homes and gardens in England and Scotland, and we wouldn't have to worry about driving on the wrong side of the road. Each morning, after a hearty English breakfast, we would clamber aboard a bus, where my biggest challenge was trying not to fall asleep while our guide, David, a former geography teacher, ran through his spiel. We toured Kent, Sussex, Harrowgate, Stourhead, Salisbury, Beaulieu, Cumbria, the Cotswolds, Stratford-Upon-Avon, Worcestershire, Winchester, Hadrian's Wall, Gretna, Edinburgh, St. Andrews and York. We wandered through rose gardens and Tudor palaces. We visited the Royal Yacht, *Britannia*, and gawked at the narrow twin beds slept in by Prince Philip and Her Majesty the Queen. We ate haggis, fish and chips, Scottish beef, salmon and saddle of lamb, trifle, sticky pudding, and crumpets with clotted cream and strawberry jam, all washed down with cups of milky English tea.

In England, I could feel myself growing stronger. I was still depressed, but I now had enough stamina to get through the arbitration over my dismissal back in Toronto.

The arbitration was public. After nearly two years of imposed silence, I had yearned for this chance, finally, to speak freely. The union sent two officials, a lawyer and an articling student. The company sent six lawyers and senior executives. Anticipating we'd be out-gunned, I invited a few friends for moral support. Ten showed up. "Are they selling tickets in the lobby?" the arbitrator joked.

"Yes, they are," replied my friend Joyce.

The arbitrator had the power to reinstate me, but given the poisoned relationship the likelihood of reinstatement was close to zero. But before we could even get started, she announced that she wanted to attempt confidential mediation over my dismissal before trying public arbitration. My friends were politely ejected.

To my dismay, I discovered I had no right to speak. Instead, I sat there like a lump, listening to the two warring parties, my employer and my union, talk about me as though I wasn't there. For the next eleven hours, the arbitrator-turned-mediator shuttled back and forth between the company and the union (and me) trying to hammer out a deal. By evening, I was exhausted, dehydrated and so cold I was trembling, but I told the arbitrator that I could not agree to what had been proposed. She stared disbelievingly at me and said she would leave the offer open for seven days.

For me, a big principle was at stake: an automatic gag order. Keeping silent for the rest of my life was a deal-breaker. I knew that if I simply took the cash and agreed not to speak, ever, about what had happened, I might never recover. But how could I justify walking away from so much money when I was jobless, unable to write and still had two boys to put through university? This was more than my decision alone. As my psychiatrist had put it, four lives were involved.

Ben talked it through with me, as always. He urged me to turn down the money. Sam had one question. "Is it a lot-lot? Like, more than you'll ever make in your life?" I admitted it was a ton of money. "Don't take it," Sam said. By that point, Norman had found a good job developing software to protect the electric-utility grid from terrorist attacks. In his deadpan way, he said, "A lifelong gag order doesn't sound so bad to me." Then he quickly added, "Don't take it."

Gigi had already said that any deal conditional on a gag order was a bad deal. Dad, now eighty-eight, made it unanimous.

For some people, principle is paramount. In accusing the Ford Motor Company of stealing his design of the intermittent windshield wiper, Robert Kearns lost his job, savings, marriage and, temporarily, his sanity. At first, the automaker ignored him. Then it offered to settle for two hundred and fifty thousand dollars and, later, for $1 million. On the eve of trial, Ford offered $30 million. Kearns turned that down, too, when Ford still balked at acknowledging him as the lawful inventor. In the end, he got the acknowledgment *and* $28.9 million from Ford and Chrysler.

Although I was improving, I still took meds. Twice a day, I swallowed a round, electric-blue, 100-milligram pill of Wellbutrin, my fourth antidepressant. Occasionally, I popped an anxiety pill, too. The side effects included dry mouth and dry eyes, and now there was a new one: heart palpitations.

My psychiatrist began urging me to abandon the struggle. "Your tenacious will to win is going to blind you to family and other relationships."

I nodded. But I still felt I couldn't walk away.

The following week, Dr. Menchions gave me another well-timed nudge. "I think you have a conflict of interest. You are staying sick because you have to convince them that you are sick. You do not want to stay sick to prove your point. That's a betrayal of yourself."

His words jolted me. For months, I had been trying so hard to prove I was honest about being sick that I had forgotten about getting better. I had been sleepwalking through my illness. Now I suddenly woke up. At my next session, I told Dr. Menchions I wanted to stop taking antidepressants. He suggested I wait a few more weeks. I did and then, under his supervision, I began reducing my dosage of Wellbutrin.

Getting off antidepressants is difficult. Even with my doctor's help, it was terribly hard to wean myself. My mood plunged and, once again, I began weeping over every little thing. At home I became unbearable, again. I either withdrew or flew into rages, and later wallowed in guilt. My narcissism returned. For instance, Ben's decision to spend his first year of university abroad at Herstmonceux Castle in East Sussex, England, felt like a betrayal, as though he were trying to get as far away from me as possible (even though I was the one who had pushed for the castle option in the first place.) I took it personally that he chose to leave the day before my birthday.

Joan Didion wrote about the power of grief to derange the mind. The day of my son's departure, I ricocheted between sadness and rage. First, my eyes filled with tears of despair. Then I became angry. At 11 A.M., Ben, who hadn't finished packing, was still asleep. In fact, both boys were still in bed. I stormed up the stairs, flung open their doors and began screaming. As teenagers, *they* were supposed to have tantrums.

The boys shuddered awake with small groans. Abruptly I switched to kindness. *I can't ruin Ben's last day at home.* I went back downstairs to calm myself, had another silent cry and wiped my face. Then I went meekly back up to their rooms. "What would you guys like for lunch?" I asked, affecting an attitude of maternal solicitude.

"Nothing," Sam said sleepily. "Me and Ben are going to a movie."

I let the bad grammar pass. A few weeks earlier, I had urged Ben to do something special with his brother before leaving for another continent. But I didn't mean they should go to the movies *the very day Ben was leaving*. I'm not sure what chemicals were unbalancing my brain. In a flash, I became enraged, again. I stomped off to the kitchen and began banging pots around. I was disintegrating, but I had to cook.

It's Ben's last meal at home.

I crept back upstairs to ask if I could go with them to the movies. "You won't like it," said Sam kindly. Then he uttered two magic words: "Seth Rogen." Sam knew I was no fan of the star of *Knocked Up* and *Superbad*. Glumly, I went back downstairs. I cried some more. I glanced again at the clock and fell apart. There wasn't enough time to make lunch *and* get to the movies. *And* I was losing my eldest son. I started sobbing.

"We don't need to eat first," Ben said quietly, coming into the kitchen.

"We don't want you to come," said Sam, nicely, trailing Ben.

It turns out the movie excursion was a ruse, and I was ruining it. Sam had planned to sneak out and buy me a birthday present. I was clueless. I only knew I was so nuts I was willing to watch Seth Rogen.

"Make Ben some sandwiches for the airport," I snapped at Sam.

Without a word, my younger son made a stack of peanut butter and tuna sandwiches. Meanwhile Ben packed, weighed his suitcases and repacked. I stood by helplessly. I had wanted a Hallmark-happy farewell. Instead, I was going berserk and making everyone miserable.

And then, suddenly, Ben was … gone. He would not email home for days.

The next day, Sam set his alarm. He was now without an ally in the struggle to cope with a crazy mom. He came down to the kitchen in boxer shorts, rubbing his eyes. Then he whipped up a birthday feast for me: orange juice; milky tea; sliced peaches and bananas atop unsweetened yogurt; bacon; toasted cornbread; and an omelet of Havarti cheese, shredded chicken, Worcestershire sauce and maple syrup.

He peered anxiously at the tawny-hued omelet. "Is it good?"

I took a bite. It was very special. "Delicious," I said. "Let's share it."

Sam suggested—surprise—going to a movie with me. I proposed, instead of the Seth Rogen flick, a film called *Mongol*, a Russian-Mongolian-

Kazakhstan-German co-production about Genghis Khan.

"It has subtitles," I warned.

Sam said he *loved* subtitles.

To my surprise, he enjoyed the film, leaning forward for a better look at every slash-and-burn scene. The movie recounted the story of the young Genghis Khan, who as a boy was kidnapped and forced to wear a heavy wooden cangue around his neck and hands. He was beaten and tortured, shot in the back with an arrow and watched helplessly as his father died of poison.

But he never gave up.

Suddenly I realized I *was* losing my mind: I was feeling sorry for Genghis Khan.

A few weeks later, it was time for another arbitration. Gigi came to Toronto to help again. Norman took the day off and this time Sam came, too. It was his summer vacation and, incorrigibly, I hoped he might learn something from the experience. It was supposed to be a public hearing, but again, the arbitrator proposed a confidential mediation. After several hours of negotiations, I again turned the deal down.

"You are going to lose the money and be tied up for five or six years," the union rep warned. He was apoplectic with rage.

Then union lawyer jumped out of his chair and wagged a finger at me. "If you let this deal fall through, you are insane!"

I was too startled to speak. Calling me "insane" was not very tactful, all things considered. It was another pivotal moment. Suddenly I realized I didn't give a rat's ass what management or the union or any arbitrator thought because none of them cared whether I would be under a gag order for the rest of my life.

We negotiated for hours. The mediation got nowhere. "I'm afraid we're going to have to go to arbitration," I said wearily to the arbitrator. "After all, I'm insane, right?"

He had the grace to look embarrassed. "No, you're not insane," the arbitrator said. "You are not insane."

We all went home.

And so there were more mediations and arbitrations. I estimated that by now the newspaper had spent at least one hundred thousand dollars on legal proceedings. Just before the tenth hearing, by coincidence, I took my last little blue pill of Wellbutrin. Now completely off meds, I waited for the tears, the familiar swamp of depression. Nothing happened. I seemed to be okay.

Over the phone that weekend, Gigi tried to prepare me for the next arbitration. She talked about happiness. She said I didn't need external approval to be happy. It was another epiphany. Suddenly I knew Gigi was right. Happiness didn't come from my work, my status or my workplace. It came from within.

Four days later, when my sister arrived for the arbitration, the chemistry in the meeting room seemed changed. I was no longer a defeated, depressed person. And I must have radiated something because by mid-afternoon, the company had caved. The gag order was over. My sole concession was this: I promised to keep the terms of the settlement confidential, which is why I can't disclose the amount of money I received.

Until the very end, the company tried to keep one more clause a secret. I insisted it be public, or the deal was off. Please indulge me here while I quote it in full: "The Employer acknowledges that the Grievor was ill and unable to attend work from June 11, 2007 to November 13, 2007 for that reason."

When the arbitrator hurried back, brandishing that last clause in writing, I exhaled. Two years had elapsed since the Dawson shooting. A weight was lifted from my shoulders. I *had* been truthful when I said I was sick.

By mid-afternoon, it was all over. Gigi and I huddled in the hallway. "You got everything you wanted!" she whispered excitedly. I faxed a copy of the proposed settlement to my lawyer, the one whom I had hired months earlier to advise me. He was pleasantly shocked.

"It's pretty much your blueprint," he said. "Sign it."

The union rep was still pacing in the hallway. When I told him I would accept the deal, he was so nervous I might change my mind he slapped the paperwork up against the wall and yanked a pen from his pocket. I signed it, right there in the hall.

I wanted to dance a jig, but I kept a straight face. Gigi had trained me in the art of negotiation. When you win big, she always warned, you do not smile. You do not chuckle. You look inscrutable.

"Aren't you happy?" my union chairperson said, grouchily. "You got everything you wanted."

We all rode silently in the elevator together. Then Gigi and I waved goodbye to all the lawyers and the union reps, and went down into the subway station. Once safely inside a subway car, I waited for the doors to close. Then I turned to my little sister.

"Can I smile now?" I asked meekly.

"Yes. You can."

CHAPTER 27

Eat Bread. Butter, Too

It was over. I would never again have to go into the newsroom. I would never have to meet with anyone whose title included the two words: "human resources." I would never have to talk to my Manulife "intervention specialist." I was done being intervened with.

My sister and I called Dad right away. "Very good. Very good," he said proudly. "I knew you would win."

Gigi hurried back to Montreal to take care of him. That night she phoned me to report that the *Globe* had just called her offering a half-price subscription. Then the *Globe* called Colleen with a similar offer. "No thanks," she said.

"May I ask why?"

"Because I'm Jan Wong's cousin."

"That'll do it," the telemarketer said, laughing.

Two weeks later, a big, fat check landed in my account. I looked at the sum and grinned. A month later, I decided for both financial and psychological reasons that I wanted to cash out my accrued pension. I had serious doubts about the long-term survival of my newspaper. And even if the *Globe* did beat the odds, when I turned sixty-five I didn't want to receive anything marked with the name of my former employer. So I processed the paperwork and was still in cash three days later when stock markets around the world crashed and the economy went into the biggest decline since the Great Depression. I watched as some of the best newspapers across North America downsized, shuttered bureaus and filed for bankruptcy protection.

It was the worst time to look for a job in journalism. So I didn't. Instead, I savored how wonderful it was to wake up in the morning (as opposed to the middle of the night) and contemplate a new day. I began to gain a bit more weight. Happily, I could still squeeze into size-two jeans, but I stopped looking gaunt. I no longer felt like running away all the time. I practiced my flute. I cheered Sam at his hockey games. I chatted over Skype with Ben at Herstmonceux Castle.

Now that I was no longer severely depressed, I had another epiphany. Just as my self-esteem was not tied to external approval, my happiness did not depend on gathering more berries. Even with a vastly swollen bank account, shopping therapy suddenly lost its attraction.

At the same time, I began to consider the price of berries in general. It occurred to me that many of us might be able to spend less time stressed at work while spending even less money at the mall. That's because in real terms food prices have plunged 75 percent over the last thirty years, due to globalization, government subsidies and soaring productivity. Before 1952, Americans spent 20 percent of their income on food. They now spend 5.6 percent on food, the lowest percentage of any society in history. But instead of enjoying additional leisure time or saving the surplus for a rainy day, everyone began spending even more on *stuff*. We now discard shoes, clothing, toys, furniture and electronic gadgets at a faster rate than ever before, according to Juliet Schor, a Boston College sociologist who researches consumer trends.

To keep frantically shopping, people began working longer and longer hours, and they borrowed more, too. Yet as Bill Bryson noted in his memoir *The Life and Times of the Thunderbolt Kid*, increased consumption did not make Americans any happier. By the late 1950s, the middle class had "pretty much everything they had ever dreamed of, so increasingly there was nothing much to do with their wealth but buy more and bigger versions of things they didn't truly require."

What if I consciously dropped out of Consumer Nation? Could I live on less? Could I liberate myself from the dopamine-seeking shop-'til-you-drop syndrome? Exactly how many roots and berries, not to mention chunky green sofas, did I need to be happy? How much is enough?

Obviously, in the poorest countries on Earth—the bottom 25 percent of the world—a minimum amount of wealth is required for survival and subsistence. But beyond that, it turns out there is virtually no relationship between money and happiness. In an astonishing finding that has been replicated many times, researchers have found no link between gross national product, per capita income, and levels of happiness.

Daniel Gilbert, a Harvard psychologist, claims that anyone earning $20,000 a year in a developed country would be ecstatic with a seven-fold increase to $140,000. And his research shows that someone making $140,000 a year would be happier, too, with a fifty-fold increase to $7 million—but not fifty *times* happier. Gilbert calls this the "declining marginal utility" of wealth. Simply put, you'd be really happy if you went from subsistence to abundance, and happy—but not all that happy—if you went from abundance to, well, more abundance. Consider that in the first case, more money means the difference between taking the bus and owning a car, between Kraft Dinner and a steak dinner. In the second case, you'd still be driving a car, a fancier one, but you'd be stuck in the same traffic as the guy with the cheaper car. And you'd still be eating steak, maybe a more expensive cut—if you weren't on a low-cholesterol diet because you had already indulged in too much steak.

If there's virtually no relationship between money and happiness in developed countries, I wondered, how depressing is unforced frugality? I decided to find out in one of the most expensive cities on earth. *Publisher's Weekly* wanted to interview me about my Beijing book, but my U.S. publisher had no budget to fly me to New York. Perhaps I could pay my own way and do it on the cheap. On the Internet I found a seat-sale for off-peak departures. That was no problem. My entire life was now off-peak. As part of my pared-down lifestyle, I unearthed my faded, college-era L.L.Bean backpack. (An unexpected bonus: I felt young again!)

Once I was so busy I'd race to the airport at the last minute. Now I arrived a leisurely one hour early. "We close flights one hour in advance now," said the unsmiling agent when I tried to check in.

My blood pressure held steady.

"Well, then what?" the new me said pleasantly.

Maybe it was my Zen approach, or maybe it was because I had no luggage to check (also part of my new Zen approach), but the agent relented. Handing me a boarding pass, she told me to run to the gate. I was so Zen by then that I merely strolled. As I passed Starbucks, I decided against a reflexive four-dollar latte. On board the plane, I accepted a complimentary cup of caffeine-free apple juice and fell blissfully asleep, waking only when we landed at LaGuardia Airport.

Even as a penny-pinching student at Columbia, I had always taken a cab from the airport. Now I bought a seven-day New York transit pass for twenty-five dollars from a kiosk in the terminal. My niece Alisha had advised me the M60 bus would take me straight from LaGuardia to her Columbia dorm. I waited three minutes, marginally longer than I would have stood in line for a cab.

"How are you?" the friendly bus driver boomed. "Would you like a free newspaper, ma'am?" He gestured behind him to a pristine stack of *New York Daily News*. I couldn't believe it. Free was great. Then I realized free was not great for my industry. Correction: my *former* industry. It no longer was my problem, so I helped myself to a copy. Inside the newspaper, I found a coupon for a 15-percent discount at Macy's.

I soon began noticing how many things in life were free, and not just the floor of my niece's college dorm. At a coffee shop the next day, I read a discarded *New York Times*. I went to the free Friday evening at the Museum of Modern Art, snagging one of the last timed (and complimentary) tickets to an exhibit featuring Van Gogh's *Starry Night*. I listened to a free concert at the Juilliard School. I attended a Sunday morning service at Riverside Church so I could hear the magnificent carillon donated by the late John D. Rockefeller, Jr.

I zipped all over the five boroughs in search of bargain eats. Each time I went through a subway turnstile, I swear I felt a squirt of dopamine. (I *loved* getting my money's worth on the transit pass.) I sampled Korean barbecue in midtown, Sichuan noodles in Flushing, a deli sandwich on the Upper West Side. I also dined at good restaurants—Aquavit, Les Halles—where, by ordering a main *plat* and skipping dessert, I ate very well at near-budget prices and still had enough for a generous tip.

At the Metropolitan Museum of Art, where entry is pay-what-you-will (but twenty dollars is strongly suggested), I wondered if I had the nerve to pay less. And how would it feel? I put down five dollars.

"The suggested admission is twenty dollars," the ticket seller said automatically.

"I know. I want to pay five."

Without changing expression, the ticket seller took my money and gave me a ticket. I felt only a tiny bit sheepish. I told myself I was unemployed now. And I assuaged my conscience by staying only one hour.

The last time I went to the Metropolitan Opera, I had bought the most expensive ticket. This time I bought the cheapest. The great Seiji Ozawa was conducting Tchaikovsky's *The Queen of Spades*. My seat, which cost one-tenth what I had spent last time, was in the nosebleed section. I could hear the orchestra and soloists just fine. But unless the performers waved their arms, it was sometimes hard to figure out which little pin-figure was actually singing. Still, this time I didn't cry.

On the appointed day, I met the editor from *Publisher's Weekly* at Jean Georges, a three-starred Michelin restaurant, which offered a three-course lunch for twenty-eight dollars. I ordered young garlic soup with sautéed frog legs for my first course, followed by roasted sweetbreads with fragrant pickled peach, wild arugula and pink peppercorn. Then I settled back in the midnight-blue velvet banquette to enjoy myself.

To my horror, the glamorous (and stick thin) editor who was interviewing me waved off the breadbasket. "I never eat bread," she said.

"Neither do I," the waiter purred as he retreated. "It makes you full."

"I thought that was the point of eating," I said, summoning him back. I helped myself to thick slices of artisanal baguette and house-made sourdough. I slathered on sweet butter. I chewed a mouthful and savored the moment. A new motto for the rest of my life suddenly popped into my head: "Eat bread. Butter, too."

I do realize how blessed I was to have been able to shop, travel and eat my way around the world without filing for personal bankruptcy. I now understand that the biggest luxury good of all is not foie gras, but freedom. I'm also keenly aware that many others with depression haven't the means to dull the pain the way I did. Still, my trip to New York taught me that the geographic cure did not require spending lavishly. Despite dropping an average of just forty dollars a day on three meals, entertainment and transportation, I was enjoying myself immensely. I realized that the key was savoring life as it unfolded. For the first time in my life, I was rushing exactly nowhere.

On my way home, after my plane landed in Toronto, I experimented with taking public transit from the airport. The trip would involve three buses. Would it take all day and be horribly crowded? In fact, each time the transfer was efficient, and on each bus I managed to get a seat. The total journey along city streets took only half an hour longer than an airport limo on the congested expressway. And it cost only $2.25 instead of fifty dollars.

By now I seemed to be well past the phase of half-recovery, the stage of anhedonia where nothing seems enjoyable. I was completely off antidepressants, but was still seeing Dr. Menchions. On this trip to New York, I was pleased and relieved that I had handled all the logistics myself. I figured that as the strife with the *Globe* had ended, everything henceforth would be roses and sunshine. Right? Wrong. I still wasn't able to write. When I attempted to write this book, the first draft was unusable.

My depression, which lasted two years, was three times as long as the average episode—and I still wasn't completely back to normal. "Everyone has a unique way of coming out of depression," Dr. Menchions told me. "You had all kinds of assaults on your mind. You were accused of malingering. Someone who didn't work as closely with the mind might not be as bad."

Recovery is different for everyone, and not necessarily a straight line. Getting over a depression is not the same as getting over a cold. With depression, there can be many mini-relapses on the way to wellness. Everything's going swimmingly and then suddenly you have a minor setback—or two. You are constantly checking in with your psyche. Are you feeling sad, justifiably, because something bad has happened to you? Or are you feeling sad because you're depressed? Friends kept inquiring if I was okay. I honestly didn't know what to say. I felt much better, but what was *okay*? Diagnosing wellness after a depression is as problematic and elusive as diagnosing the illness in the first place. On the spectrum between sickness and health, when are you finally out of the woods?

"Emergence is usually slow, and people stop at various stages of it," Solomon writes in *The Noonday Demon.* "You don't get over breakdowns quickly or easily. Things go on being bumpy."

I know this much: once you've lost your mind, you never feel secure again. The specter of depression—that stunning 50-percent relapse rate—is ever present. Perhaps it is a bit like being in remission from cancer. Even after you've beaten it, you worry the disease will return. Sometimes I felt as though I was still struggling upstream and that if I ever stopped paddling, I would get sucked back into the vortex. I was surprised how little it took to push me back down. Some people face a lifetime of depressive episodes. Anxiously I asked my psychiatrist whether he thought I was vulnerable to a relapse. I was inexpressibly relieved when he shook his head. "Your depression was caused by your situation at work. You'll build up calluses."

Five months after I signed my deal with the *Globe,* I attended a black-tie fundraiser for Toronto's public library system. I was apprehensive because it was the kind of literati event that attracted journalists. As body armor, I again donned my expensive black cocktail dress. At the pre-dinner reception, a radio journalist I knew approached me. "They wanted to get rid of you from the get-go," she said, sipping her wine. "From what I've seen, they didn't support you at all." She scanned my face for signs (I suppose) of ravages.

I wanted to protest: *No, no. That wasn't it at all.* But how could I summarize the two worst years of my life in cocktail-party chatter? I was still groping for the right words when I realized that she had already moved on.

Get rid of you. The words stung. I almost burst into tears, right next to the silent-auction tables. That surprised me. I thought I no longer cared what others thought. Dr. Menchions was right. I needed to build up calluses. But building up calluses first required getting blisters that hurt. Whenever someone asked what I did for a living, or where I worked, I suddenly felt self-conscious, vulnerable and defensive. I would say that I wrote. It didn't help when they asked, "Full time?"

Once upon a time I had the world at my feet. Now that I was home, alone and unemployed, many people, especially other journalists, viewed me as someone not worth bothering about. At least, that's how I saw it on the days when I felt down, when I forgot about my epiphanies and my newfound frugality and freedom. Without my influential perch at the newspaper, it seemed that I no longer had anything to offer others, no network, no tidbits of gossip, no prestige, not even a potential job contact.

All societies have to some extent focused on work. But modern Western culture is the first to hold that a "meaningful existence must invariably pass through the gate of remunerative employment," says Alain de Botton, author of *The Pleasures and Sorrows of Work*. Dominique Browning, who lost her job as editor of *House & Garden* when the magazine abruptly closed down in 2007, was surprised that nobody seemed to have time for her anymore. A former friend did get in touch, only to gloat, "You've lost your power! Now I can say anything I want to you."

At that library fundraiser, like many authors, I had been assigned to a corporate table. I found mine and managed to introduce myself to the other guests. The host smiled awkwardly. A beat later, after I sat down, I understood why. I was at the wrong table. I stood up feeling stupid and worthless. When you've had a mental illness, you assume every snafu is your fault. At the time, it did not occur to me that perhaps the volunteer who pointed me to that table had erred.

A week later, someone from the fundraiser called. She said I was the successful bidder of some silent-auction items and had neglected to pay before I left. Apparently I had bid eighty dollars for two T-shirts and a fleece jacket. I had no memory of bidding on them. In my new frugality mode, I thought I had successfully stopped shopping. Was my mind playing tricks on me? Trying to hide how upset I was, I found my credit card and recited the number to her.

Ten minutes later, the same woman called back. It had all been a mistake. I began laughing with relief. I blathered on about how she had given me such a shock. I had been depressed, you see, which had affected my memory and that's why I hadn't protested, even though I didn't remember bidding on the clothing at all.

There was silence, followed by an effusive apology.

People don't like to hear about depression, so I finally stopped babbling. After I hung up the phone, I smiled. Perhaps I *was* out of the woods. If you can hang in there long enough, depression eventually capitulates.

"Mysterious in its coming, mysterious in its going, the affliction runs its course and one finds peace," Styron writes.

CHAPTER 28

Roses

To thank my friend Joyce and three other women for their support throughout my illness, I invited them to dinner on Valentine's Day. On my mahogany dining table (newly refinished for $1,900 during my berry-gathering phase), I set out heirloom Coalport china and vintage lace-edged napkins (the latter also purchased during the same phase).

I once whipped up dinner parties in ninety minutes, but I hadn't fully bounced back because the preparation for this one took hours. By the middle of the afternoon, I had to lie down. My memory was still problematic. I had to write down the most obvious tasks:

> *Set out chilled butter*
> *Bread plates*
> *Pepper grinder*
> *Matches to light candles*

I bought four bouquets of tulips, roses and ginger flowers, one for each friend to take home after dinner. Massed on the table, they looked stunning. Another motto for the rest of my life: you can never have too many roses.

The women arrived bearing champagne truffles and wine. While they sat around my kitchen table nibbling on foie gras toasts, I prepared a peppercorn-crusted filet of beef. Once I finished cooking the main course, we moved into the dining room. Norman sat at the head of the table, enjoying his Valentine's date with five women.

"You know those three boys who were pushed in the subway station yesterday?" said Joyce. She added that one of the injured was the son of the *Globe's* editor-in-chief. I was shocked. After my dinner guests left, I checked the Internet and learned that the boy would require surgery on one of his feet. The accused, a forty-seven-year-old man named Adenir DeOliveira, had been charged with three counts of attempted murder and two accounts of assault. A *Toronto Star* story reported:

> *Duty counsel Al Hart asked that DeOliveira be given access to three*

prescription drugs: Effexor, used to treat anxiety and depression; Lorazepam, used to relieve the short-term symptoms of anxiety; and Seroquel, used to treat symptoms of schizophrenia as well as acute manic episodes associated with bipolar disorder.

A psychiatric evaluation has also been ordered for DeOliveira.

I shut off my computer and shivered. The subway assault rekindled memories of my own moment on the platform, when I had contemplated jumping. And like the accused, I had been prescribed two of the same drugs, Effexor and lorazepam, the tranquilizer sold as Ativan.

I suddenly felt dizzy. I went into the kitchen to wash my china dishes. As I plunged my arms into the hot, soapy water, I realized that one of the worst aspects of depression is that so many people don't believe you. But the subway assault on the three boys had been so dramatic, horrifying and public that no one would ever doubt that the boy who had been physically injured would also suffer emotionally. His visible scars would always remind those around him what had happened. If in future he had a phobia about using the subway, no one would tell him to snap out of it. He would rightfully receive abundant sympathy.

Given the list of prescription drugs requested by the defence lawyer, I assumed the alleged perpetrator was mentally ill. As an invisible affliction, always hard to quantify, mental illness elicits far less understanding. Certainly there is zero sympathy for those who hurt innocents. Seven months later, DeOliveira appeared in Ontario Superior Court and pleaded not guilty to three counts of attempted murder and three counts of assaulting transit employees. His lawyer said he was not criminally responsible for his alleged actions because of his mental illness.

For two years, I thought the sofa in my doctor's office was made of green leather. The other day I noticed it was in fact dark red leather. I had always thought the plants in his office were real. Now I noticed they were artificial. It made me wonder anew about the power of depression to bend reality.

As I got better, I began to fear my doctor would ditch me. I didn't feel at all ready to end my sessions. One day I asked him, "Does this mean I have to stop seeing you?"

"Oh, no," Dr. Menchions said. "There's still lots of work to do. When you're depressed, everything gets distorted, including your sense of self."

That was a relief, but his words also disheartened me. *Lots of work to do.* My psychiatrist explained there would be post-traumatic stress. He said that my confidence would require rebuilding. He warned that I had to work on my family relationships. I also needed to get back to writing—I still wasn't able to write. And, no small matter, I had to figure out what I would do to earn a living.

For more than a year, I'd been seeing Dr. Menchions once a week, sometimes more frequently. Now as I improved, he began scheduling my appointments at two-week intervals. Then he tried a three-week gap, but that felt too unnerving. We temporarily went back to two weeks. A month later, he tried a three-week interval, this time with success. I'm now down to once a month and I can foresee a time when I can stop going altogether.

As I write this, my Costco daffodils are blooming for the third year. Every time I look at them, I have to smile. I think about my family doctor's wise cure. I think about how Norman and the boys chose the red and yellow hues when I could not make a decision. In two days, Ben is flying back home after a year in England. My psychiatrist explained that his desire to separate from me is natural and healthy, so I no longer feel bad about that. I'm glad my son has taken flight.

When I was in the United Kingdom on a book tour this spring, I took a few days to visit Ben at Herstmonceux Castle. I had been reading *Mrs. Dalloway* and I noticed that my train from London took me past the River Ouse, where Virginia Woolf committed suicide. At the castle, I audited a few of my son's lectures. One of his professors lectured on, yes, *Mrs. Dalloway*.

Life kept playing jokes on me. On my second day, at lunch in the great hall, I set down my tray and greeted the kid on my left. A moment later, I realized he was the son of the *Globe*'s publisher. Don't worry. I was the soul of discretion. But what are the odds of that?

After Ben returned from his year in England, we went on a midnight excursion to a park near our home. He wanted to practise one-armed chin-ups on the monkey bars, and invited me to tag along. Had I still had a job, I would have been asleep. But I went with him into the balmy spring night, leaving the front door unlocked. Ben did his chin-ups and then we returned to a darkened house.

Someone had locked us out. I peered through the sidelights, and rang the bell. Sam eventually let us in.

"Auntie Gigi called," he said.

My sister and I now talked by phone all the time, sometimes twice a day, even late at night. I was in the living room and had just started telling her about my excursion to the park when I was startled by a loud bang. Someone was rapping on the window with a metal flashlight. A man. A *stranger*.

Alarmed, I put down the phone and shouted for reinforcements. "Someone's in the driveway!" Ben was instantly at my side. Sam arrived a moment later, gripping a baseball bat. (Norman, who was sick, was asleep.)

Through the sidelights, I spied a uniform, then a patch on a sleeve: *Toronto Police.* I opened the door a crack.

"We received a report of a break-in," the police officer said.

Confused, I explained about my son's midnight chin-ups and described how we had been locked out. I stopped in mid-sentence and gaped. Half a dozen cops were swarming over our front lawn. Three others were searching my neighbor's bushes. Three more were circling around from the back of our house. Six squad cars were parked in front, lights flashing. As I stared in disbelief, I heard the officer at our door calling off the search.

"Have a good evening," he said politely, backing away.

The police officers left as silently as they had come. As the squad cars drove away, I stood there dumbfounded. Who had called 911? And why would a possible break-and-enter merit a Hollywood-thriller takedown?

An hour later, it clicked. Our address was still on the elite 911 list. I had forgotten all about it, but two years and eight months later, the police had not. Neither had Sam, who still kept his baseball bat tucked under the bookcase in his bedroom.

My younger son is doing fine now. To his delight, he's now taller than Norman. And last year, after nearly failing math, he took a summer course and aced it. "I can't believe it," he said at dinner the other night. "I've *doubled* my math mark. And Mom, the biology teacher said I've really improved." Recently, the school sent congratulations because Sam's average finally exceeded 75 percent—high enough to get him off academic probation.

As a parent, I have always wanted to prepare my sons for what lies ahead in life. And while I'm not sure I would have chosen to impart quite so lurid a lesson, I know they have learned resilience from me. You can pay for all the skiing and piano lessons you want, but in the end, a child who has watched a parent solve a seemingly insurmountable life problem gains immeasurably in wisdom, sensitivity and self-confidence. Adversity made us stronger.

As the American poet Maya Angelou notes, a diamond is the result of extreme pressure and time. Norman is a diamond. He has stuck by me through extreme pressure and time. And he's still trying to humor the insane. The other day, he went uncomplainingly to the movies in the middle of the week. He had just gotten home from work when I announced we had to see a movie that very night because a free pass from a cereal box was about to expire. (The new frugality, you understand.)

We saw *State of Play*, about a Washington reporter who uncovers corporate mayhem and murder. I suppose I wanted to see a movie about a newspaper for the same reason people read old love letters long after the affair is over. The film wasn't very realistic. Russell Crowe, a sartorially challenged investigative reporter, misses his deadline by, oh, five hours, *but he still makes the front page!* Even while suspending disbelief, I felt I was watching a nearly extinct breed: Hollywood's last hero journalist, armed with an old-fashioned notepad and extra ballpoint pens.

To be honest, I hadn't been happy in recent years at the newspaper. Everywhere journalists have lost control over their stories, and I was no different. Editors today want quicker and quicker turnarounds with no time for serious reporting. Too many assignments are tasteless or shallow. Still, I miss the thrill of the chase, the deadlines, the scoops, the instant gratification of the daily byline.

The most precious gift to come out of this painful episode has been my relationship with my sister. In the years after our mother's death, she excised me from her life. At the time, I was angry. The worst part was I didn't even realize what a loss this was, or would have been. And then I got sick. Despite our estrangement, my sister flew to the rescue. She shored up my disintegrating family. She prodded me to raid my office. She listened to me cry. Okay, she took me shopping at La-Z-Boy, but she also drove through the night to make every key mediation and arbitration. Whenever I crumpled, she became my spine.

We weren't best friends before. We are now. If I had not had this crisis, we might have stayed apart for the rest of our lives. We now understand each other much better. I listen to her advice. I respect and admire her. And I try not to be so selfish and self-centered. As Dad grows ever more frail, I know now that I cannot make the same mistake I made with Mom. I try to visit him frequently. I take him south when the weather turns cold. And I phone him as often as I can although he remains as taciturn as ever.

"Dad, how are you?"

"I'm okay! I'm okay! Do you want to talk to Gigi?"

My life is full with writing, friends and music. I've freelanced as a radio host, written some magazine columns and started a new career as a journalism professor, passing on my experience to the next generation. To make a point about the reliability of eyewitnesses and to teach them to be ready at any moment to jump on a story, I punk'd the students in one of my classes.

I hired an actress to burst into my classroom and impersonate a maid from my minimum-wage series. And then I made them write up the incident on deadline. What color were her eyes? How tall was she? Exactly what did she say? When a few figured out she wasn't for real, I gave them bonus points for skepticism.

I love my students. I make them report and write and report and re-write until they plead for respite. I teach them basic rules: "Show, don't tell." "Good quotes up high." They actually take my advice to heart. Teaching gives me great satisfaction, which surprises me. Even after I left my newspaper, I thought the only way I could be happy in journalism was by chasing my own stories.

Shockingly, except for the chase and the bylines, I do not miss my workplace at all. But I have to start using the past tense. I don't know why, even at the end of this journey, I keep slipping up and referring to it as "my" newspaper. I have to keep reminding myself to stop saying "we" when I mention the *Globe*. Is it mere force of habit? Or does it mean I haven't yet purged the toxins from my system? Despite the bit about reporters being the enduring carpet and all that, I was just an employee. I only worked there. I now realize it was never "my" newspaper.

It seems my timing was exquisite. Like the stunt man diving through the plate-glass window right before the building explodes, I got out in the nick of time. Four months after the big fat check landed, the *Globe* announced a massive downsizing. The newsroom rumor was my settlement had bankrupted the paper. When colleagues called to ask, I told them unfortunately I couldn't confirm or deny anything—and then we all enjoyed a good chuckle.

Then one day the publisher fired the editor-in-chief. Friends instantly phoned and emailed me with the news. I grinned. I laughed out loud. Cackling, I called my sister, who thought my euphoria so alarming that she urged me to talk to my psychiatrist. Everyone was still second-guessing me. *I* was still second-guessing myself. Was my behavior inappropriate? I asked Dr. Menchions. He smiled. "It's completely natural to feel this after what happened to you."

No one was safe at the newspaper. One day you're golden, the next day you're garbage. At least I had had time to adjust to being un-golden before I was put out with the trash. My direct report, Cathrin Bradbury, the deputy managing editor of features, was fired next and then the vice-president of human resources suddenly left. Next one of the top five managers was diagnosed with prostate cancer. Despite his health problems, he was fired, too. (He soon landed at a rival newspaper.)

A few weeks after the old editor-in-chief was sacked, the new editor-in-chief phoned me out of the blue.

"How are you?" he said.

I nearly dropped the phone. The last time I talked to John Stackhouse was in the midst of the Dawson crisis. He had been the business editor then, and the one who told me I had misconstrued my appointment as Asia-Pacific correspondent.

Now, suppressing my surprise, I tried to answer his question. *How was I?* I was launching into a medical explanation when I caught myself.

"Oh, sorry. I mean: I'm fine. Thank you. How are you?"

"No, I do want to know how you are," he said warmly.

The new editor-in-chief said he was calling to commission a 1,500-word piece to mark the fiftieth anniversary of the *Globe*'s Beijing bureau. There would be a special section with articles from every former Beijing correspondent. "It would be wonderful to have you be part of that. No one can think of the China bureau without thinking of you. On a personal level, I'd be honored to have you be part of it."

My head reeled. "I haven't written any journalism since ..."

I paused, unable to finish my sentence. I told him I'd think about it, and hung up the phone.

But I didn't call him back. In the days and weeks that followed I pushed the offer from my mind. It was all too confusing. Then a friend suggested the editor's approach might be an olive branch. That suddenly put it in another light. Peace is good—another motto for the rest of my life. A month after he first called me, I left a voice-mail message for the new editor-in-chief, telling him I'd do it.

Stackhouse emailed back right away: "I'm absolutely thrilled that you're keen to write for our bureau anniversary section. It would be bafflingly incomplete without you ... It will be a happy day for our readers to see your name in the *Globe* again."

That's how nutty the workplace can be. I'd just been paid a pile of money to go away. And now the paper wanted to pay me a tidy sum to write for them again. When the piece was published, the newspaper surprised me again by splashing my name atop the front page: "Jan Wong ... returns to the *Globe*'s Pages."

You like me? You don't like me? You like me?

Was I having a Sally-Field type relapse? Was I misperceiving reality, again? No, I wasn't. This really is the way some workplaces are.

The final, delicious frisson was a call from a telemarketer named Kevin. "The *Globe* is offering a special 40 percent off on home delivery," he said. "It only costs $23.32 a month, including tax." The deal included a twenty-five-dollar gift card of my choice for Starbucks, Indigo Books and Music or Loblaws. I did the math. My former newspaper was offering to pay *me* $1.68 a month just to read it. Unfortunately for Kevin, I was no longer in berry-gathering mode. I told him I'd think about it.

Gigi, of course, had a better answer. "You should have said, 'Well, I used to subscribe to the *Globe*. But I canceled after I stopped seeing any articles by Jan Wong.'"

"Writing is a form of therapy," Graham Greene, the novelist, wrote. "Sometimes I wonder how all those who do not write, compose or paint can manage to escape the madness, the melancholia, the panic fear which is inherent in the human situation."

For me, writing about depression was *not* therapeutic. It made me relive the worst days again and again. But the creative act of setting down words eventually created a certain distance from the source of despair. Once the record is there, written down in full, I'm finally free to purge this terrible period from my brain. I can now stop ruminating about it, over and over again. "It is only by putting it into words that I make it whole; this wholeness means that it has lost its power to hurt me," wrote Virginia Woolf, in her 1939 autobiographical essay, "A Sketch of the Past."

The therapeutic benefit begins now, after I have put this experience into words and made it whole, and the illness has been processed. There *is* comfort in structuring the chaos and the madness. The mere act of trying to explain a trauma helps defang it. Pessimism, instead of being a waste of mental energy, has a purpose. It helps you understand your relationship to the problem and provides valuable insights. Understanding offers a solution, healing and peace.

As I've said, peace is good. Looking back, it seems that I was strong and sick simultaneously. Even while I was deeply depressed, part of me was still the reporter, observing, questioning and taking on an advocacy role for mental-illness awareness. In the end, I do not regret experiencing the demon of depression. I have learned so much. In *Homage to Catalonia*, George Orwell writes about the value of a negative experience. In 1938, he went to Spain to report on the civil war. He soon joined an anti-fascist militia, a nightmarish experience that ended only when he took a (non-fatal) sniper's bullet through the throat.

Those months in the trenches "formed a kind of interregnum in my life," Orwell writes, "quite different from anything that had gone before and perhaps from anything that is to come, and they taught me things that I could not have learned in any other way."

Today we live in a culture where we define ourselves almost solely by what we *do*. I finally understand how emotionally vulnerable that makes us, especially during economic crises when so many people lose their jobs. As Socrates told the Athenians at his trial for heresy, "the unexamined life is not worth living." I had been living the unexamined life. I mistook the buoyant surface of success for happiness. And then an amazingly quick series of events stripped everything away. I was forced to learn about who I am and what really matters. That is the gift of depression: it makes you withdraw and gives you time for reflection.

People who emerge from depression often find a heightened awareness of the beauty of everyday existence. To appreciate a brilliantly sunny day, there must also be a night. I now derive joy from things I had never noticed before, had no time for, when I was racing to meet deadlines. I watch the trees unfurl their pale green leaves each spring. In late summer I see the monarch butterflies and blue herons flit through the wetlands at my friend Liz's cottage. In my garden I plant mint, tarragon, basil, parsley, purple irises, pink echinacea, orange tiger lilies, hot-pink geraniums and, yes, impatiens. Instead of wading through several newspapers a day, I read Tolstoy, Hardy, Woolf and Faulkner. In Rome—Gigi and I recently went there for a week's holiday—I taste the bliss of spaghetti tossed with fresh zucchini blossoms. In Montreal I hang out on the front stoop with Dad as he leans on his cane and puffs his cigar. I have time for life.

These days, I think I finally comprehend an ancient Chinese proverb I learned by rote many years ago when I first began studying Mandarin. *Zou ma guan hua* literally means "viewing flowers from a galloping horse." The aphorism is a gentle rebuke for a life spent in haste, for failing to take the time to appreciate the good things in life. It is the Chinese version of the English maxim: stop, and smell the roses.

I have finally dismounted the galloping horse or, to be brutally honest, the horse tossed me off. At any rate, I have now mostly recovered from the injuries caused by that fall. In future I will walk beside the horse, loosely holding its reins. I will remember that I can set my own pace in life and follow my own path. This is what it means to live an examined life. This is what it means to smell the roses.

Afterword

Many books describe lifelong struggles with recurring depression or the breakdown brought on by the loss of a loved one. Few recount a workplace depression. At first, I didn't understand why. Now, after writing this book, I finally do: gag orders.

Throughout the three years my Doubleday editor, Nita Pronovost, and I worked on the manuscript, I simultaneously had to fight ongoing battles with those who wanted to silence me. In the West, we pride ourselves on freedom of speech, freedom of expression and freedom of the press. But the hard reality is that when anyone tangles with a powerful corporation or organization, those freedoms typically vanish with any settlement agreement. Financial pressures and emotional exhaustion mean few individuals can hold out for long.

Gag orders blight our democracy. From the beginning, they were a way for the powerful to stifle dissenting opinions. The concept originated in the 1830s when the United States House of Representatives used a "gag rule" to shut down debate on slavery. Today gag orders are imposed by the courts with disconcerting frequency and, ironically, are strenuously objected to by media organizations such as *The Globe and Mail*.

Gag orders also have become virtually automatic in legal settlements between powerful institutions and powerless individuals, especially when scandal is involved. When the Catholic Church or the Boy Scouts settle sexual-abuse lawsuits for instance, victims are often silenced. Silence and shame become close companions, especially when money changes hands. The secrecy imposed by a gag order makes it harder for victims to heal, especially when they cannot confide even in those closest to them.

In my case, I faced multiple gag orders by powerful players. Each time, I fought back and won. Then, just when I thought I had cleared the last hurdle, my book publisher tried to impose a gag order, too. Out of the blue (dare I say?) Doubleday pulled the plug on this book—and then wanted me to keep the matter confidential.

Nita, my editor, had been a keystroke away from sending the manuscript to copy edit, the final stage before printing (and I have her email confirming that). Suddenly, the publisher at Doubleday notified my agent she had a problem with the manuscript. She assured him, and then me, that her concerns were not legal. Indeed, several months earlier Doubleday's libel lawyer had finished vetting the manuscript. The company had even begun taking pre-orders, advertising this book on its website with the hardcover price ($29.95), estimated number of pages (352) and publication date (May 24, 2011).

As the manuscript had not radically changed in months, I was both alarmed and confused. We met and I asked the publisher for her specific concerns. Someone at Doubleday then emailed me the manuscript back, highlighting virtually every single mention of the *Globe* (and a few of Manulife) in bright yellow. Visually, it's striking and I display a sample on my website.

A few days later we met again. The publisher said Doubleday did not want to publish the book with the *Globe* material as written, in particular the parts she called "corporate bullying." She said she thought these parts "veered from the central story of depression." I said I could not figure out how to write a book about workplace depression *without* the workplace.

We agreed to disagree.

I then asked if the *Globe* had been in touch with Doubleday. My book publisher denied that there had been any contact. Perhaps she didn't realize that I knew the *Globe*'s in-house counsel had indeed phoned Doubleday's libel lawyer a month earlier to express displeasure with an article I'd written in *Chatelaine* magazine, mentioning this upcoming memoir. The libel lawyer, of course, had immediately notified both Doubleday and me.

The *Globe* phone call turned out to be mere saber rattling. A plaintiff's first step in a libel suit is to notify the offending publication—and *Chatelaine* never heard from the *Globe*. Call me naïve, but I didn't expect a major publisher like Doubleday to lose its nerve, especially so late in the editorial process. In the final settlement, I managed to resist yet another confidentiality order (which is why I am able to write this and the above six paragraphs.)

I feared this new setback would trigger a relapse. It didn't. Of course, I was upset and disappointed, but in the normal way, being blasted out of my daily routine for two or three days. Then I got right back to work. I did ruminate over the possible reasons why my long-time publisher had bolted. That phone call from the *Globe*'s lawyer aside, did Doubleday fear the newspaper would punish it by reviewing its other authors negatively? Was the book publisher concerned about current and future business deals? Shortly after Doubleday and I parted ways, I received a general email from them (my four other books remain on their backlist) touting an "Open House Festival" of its authors, sponsored by—you guessed it—*The Globe and Mail*.

Unlike the United States or Great Britain, writers in Canada face highly concentrated media ownership. While there may be no overt censorship, there is structural censorship, meaning that the tiny number of players in itself restricts freedom of expression. In effect, a decision by any one of them not to publish can kill a book. Until now. The Internet has changed everything. Although self-publishing has existed for years, there previously was no efficient way to distribute books to the public. Today, with PayPal, and other e-commerce methods, authors can connect directly with readers. This truly is as revolutionary as the invention of the Gutenberg press.

Acknowledgments

This book is about a journey through darkness. I need to thank the many people who kept me company along the way, who held my hand, listened to me (endlessly) and provided many hugs and much wisdom. I could not have survived without them.

There is no rank to friendship, so in no particular order, I would like to thank: several stalwart, unclassifiable friends, Joyce Johnston, Linda Woronka, Cedes Iboro, Paul Yeung, Dr. James Hilton, Jeffrey Lem and Edward J. Carter; my musical friends, Lori Scopis, Holli Verkade, Nadina Jackson, Jin-shan Dai, Lynda Moon, Shelley Goodman, Emily Candy, Dr. Steve Stein and Robert Hall; my journalist friends, Talin Vartanian (who deserves special mention for reading an early draft, making excellent suggestions, urging me to self-publish when prospects for this book looked grim, expertly proofreading the final copy and even coming up with the title), Stevie Cameron, Michael D'Souza, Stephen Strauss, Dai Qing, Robert MacPherson, Geoff Stevens, Konrad Ejbich, Professor Melvin Mencher, Vivian Smith, Heather Mallick, Kamal Al-Soyalee, Maria Cheng, Jay Bryan, Elinor Reading, John Saunders, John King, Oliver Bertin, Carol Toller, Anne Ko, Sun Shuyun, Suzanne Ma and the late Val Ross; my human-rights activist friends, Cheuk Kwan, Winnie Ng and Dick Chan; my Red Bud friends, Rosabel Levitt, Brenda Shin, Sue Philpott, Elizabeth Mitchell and Cara Loncar; my go-for-a-walk, go-to-the opera, pick-some-wild-mushrooms or eat-some-Sichuan-food friends, Lori Ann Comeau, Ashley and Silvia Prime, Mary Ito, Jen Meeker, Barbara Houston, Susan Le Roy, Margaret Hepburn Valiant, Wailan Low, Alfredo Bartucci, Carolyn Scharf, Lucille Toth, Margaret Little, Inta Kierans, Peter Sawchuk, Andrew Pinto, Joseph Cheng, Angela Houpt, Bernies Mah, Cindy Bennett, Wayne McLeod, Charlotte Ip, Sylvia Soyka, Julie Jai; Christian Lloyd at Herstmonceux Castle whose lecture on *Mrs. Dalloway* opened my eyes to Virginia Woolf; my China friends, Julie Wu and William Xu, Ben Mok and Ke Naiai, Zhang Hong, Gu Weiming and Qian Qihong, Liu Xinming, Timothy Brook, Jeremy Paltiel, Catherine Sampson and James Miles, Kathy Wilhelm, Qiu Hai, Qiu Bin, Qiu Jun, Yao Yuying and the doctors in Beijing who treated my sudden deafness, Dr. Lin Zhonghui, Dr. Liu Xiangyan and Dr. Marie Shieh; my doctors in Toronto, Dr. Susan Au and Dr. Bruce Menchions; and my favorite hockey moms, Cathy Finlayson and Janet Wortsman.

I'd like to thank my twelve graduate students at Toronto's Ryerson University, the first journalism class I ever taught. They were the best an inexperienced professor could hope for—smart, fun, hard-working and inspiring in their enthusiasm and dedication: Najat Abdalhadi, Althea Manasan, Gilbert Ndikubwayezu, Candace Maracle, Liam Casey, Liem Vu, Matthew Scianitti, Wendy Gillis, Ashley Csanady, Jameson Berkow, Madeleine White and Ramya Jegatheesan.

In Fredericton, New Brunswick, Dr. Drummond Bowden alerted me to the pattern-seeking similarity between journalists and epidemiologists; and librarian Rosslyn Maston kindly read through a final draft. In Toronto, both Dr. John Chong, my cousin and a specialist in repetitive stress injuries among musicians, and Dr. Irvin Wolkoff, a psychiatrist and broadcaster, read my manuscript. They each made valuable suggestions and caught errors. Any that remain, of course, are my own.

My agent, John Pearce, was solicitous, encouraging and patient, all an agent could be for a writer who was suddenly unable to write. At Doubleday, Maya Mavjee immediately saw the importance of the book and signed me up even when it was unclear whether I could ever write again. Fortunately for her (and unfortunately for me) Maya was soon promoted up and away to a bigger publishing job in New York. Nita, my Doubleday editor, took on the arduous task of guiding a crippled writer. With grace, tact, a finely honed sense of story-telling and unlimited patience, she brought the manuscript to fruition. This book would not have happened without her. I especially thank Jonathan Webb for copy editing. His unerring ability to pinpoint sequential inconsistencies, repetitive passages and apparent contradictions vastly improved the book.

Fervent thanks to my son Ben and his friend, Shaun Bennett. Their technical knowledge helped me navigate the new world of self-publishing.

I also thank Michael Camp and Philip Lee, respectively past and current directors of the journalism department at St. Thomas University in Fredericton. As I was completing the book, they invited me to be the 2010 Visiting Irving Chair in Journalism, a fellowship that included a Woolfian room of my own (furnished, with a spectacular view of the Saint John River.) In 2011, I began a new career as a tenure-track professor of journalism there, dividing my time between Toronto and Fredericton.

Finally, I thank my family. My sister, Gigi, came to my rescue. This book is dedicated to her. My father gave his unconditional love and his unwavering belief that I would ultimately triumph—what more could any kid want? My dearest cousin-in-law, Colleen Parrish, provided strategic and caring advice throughout my ordeal and was always there for me. My husband, Norman, was unstintingly loyal and supportive. He kept our family together. Ben and Sam were so busy taking care of me they missed the chance to rebel during their teenaged years. There is still time. I can only hope I will be as understanding of them as they were of me.

Selected Bibliography

American Psychiatric Association, *Diagnostic and Statistical Manual of Mental Disorders, Fourth Edition*. Arlington, Va.: American Psychiatric Publishing, 2000.

Associated Press. "Robert Kearns, 77, Inventor of Intermittent Wipers, Dies." February 26, 2005.

Babiak, Paul and Richard D. Hare. *Snakes in Suits: When Psychopaths Go to Work*. New York: Regan Books/HarperCollins, 2006.

Beck, Melinda. "Stress So Bad It Hurts—Really." *The Wall Street Journal*, March 17, 2009, p. D1. (http://online.wsj.com/article/SB123724722718848829.html)

Bethune, Brian. "Anthropologist Lionel Tiger on Faith and Sexual Behaviour: Why Religion Comforts Us, and How Churches Act as Serotonin Factories." *Maclean's*, March 8, 2010, pp. 14-15. (http://www2.macleans.ca/2010/03/04/macleans-interview-lionel-tiger/)

de Botton, Alain. *The Pleasures and Sorrows of Work*. New York: Pantheon, 2009.

Brook, Timothy, Jérôme Bourgon and Gregory Blue. *Death By a Thousand Cuts*. Cambridge, Mass.: Harvard University Press, 2008.

Browning, Dominique. *Slow Love: How I Lost My Job, Put on My Pajamas and Found Happiness*. New York: Atlas & Company, 2010.

Bryson, Bill. *The Life and Times of the Thunderbolt Kid: A Memoir*. Toronto: Doubleday Canada, 2006.

Carson, Shelley H. "Depression, Creativity, and a New Pair of Shoes." *Psychology Today*, July 30, 2008. (http://www.psychologytoday.com/blog/life-art/200807/depression-creativity-and-new-pair-shoes)

Cunningham, Michael. *The Hours*. New York: Farrar, Straus and Giroux, 1998.

Didion, Joan. *The Year of Magical Thinking*. New York: Vintage Books, 2005.

Eckholm, Erik. "China's Crackdown on Sect Stirs Alarm Over Psychiatric Abuse." *The New York Times*, February 18, 2001. (http://www.nytimes.com/2001/02/18/world/china-s-crackdown-on-sect-stirs-alarm-over-psychiatric-abuse.html)

Elias, Marilyn. "Mental Stress Spirals With Economy: Depression Can Lead to Illness" *USA Today*, March 12, 2009, p. D1. (http://www.usatoday.com/news/health/2009-03-11-stress-poll_N.htm)

Evans, Harold. *My Paper Chase: True Stories of Vanished Times*. New York: Little, Brown, 2009.

Fitzgerald, F. Scott. "The Crack-Up," *Esquire*. Originally published as a three-part series in the February, March, and April 1936 issues of *Esquire*. On February 26, 2008, *Esquire* posted the articles online. (http://www.esquire.com/features/the-crack-up)

Flaubert, Gustave. *Madame Bovary*. New York: Dover Publications, 1996.

Freud, Sigmund. "Mourning and Melancholia," *General Psychological Theory: Papers on Metapsychology*. New York: Simon & Schuster, 1991.

Gilbert, Daniel. *Stumbling on Happiness*. Toronto: Vintage Canada, 2007.

Goode, Erica. "After Combat, Victims of an Inner War," *The New York Times*, August 1, 2009, p. A1 (http://www.nytimes.com/2009/08/02/us/02suicide.html?pagewanted=all)

Grape, Christina, et al, "Does Singing Promote Well-Being? An Empirical Study of Professional and Amateur Singers During a Singing Lesson," *Integrative Psychological & Behavioral Science,* Volume 38, Number 1, January 2002, pp. 65-74. (http://www.springerlink.com/content/960143865x16w34k/)

Jamison, Kay Redfield. *Touched With Fire: Manic-Depressive Illness and the Artistic Temperament.* New York: Simon & Schuster, 1994.
———. *An Unquiet Mind.* New York: Alfred A. Knopf, 1995.
———. *Night Falls Fast: Understanding Suicide.* New York: Vintage, 2000.

Jolly, David. "France Télécom Needs 'Radical Change' After Suicides, Report Says," *The New York Times,* March 8, 2010. (http://www.nytimes.com/2010/03/09/technology/09telecom.html?ref=francetelecomsa)

Kafka, Franz. *The Trial.* New York: Schocken Books, 1974.

Keedwell, Paul. *How Sadness Survived: The Evolutionary Basis of Depression.* Oxford: Radcliffe Publishing, 2008.

Knott, Verner J. "Depression and Smoking: Is There a Link?" press release, Canadian Psychiatric Research Foundation, March 9, 2010.

Lacasse, J.R. and Leo, J. "A Disconnect Between the Advertisements and the Scientific Literature," *Public Library of Science, Medicine* 2(12): e392, November 8, 2006. (http://www.plosmedicine.org/article/info:doi/10.1371/journal.pmed.0020392 - pmed-0020392-b14)

Lehrer, Jonah. "Depression's Upside," *The New York Times Sunday Magazine,* February 28, 2010, p. 38. (http://www.nytimes.com/2010/02/28/magazine/28depression-t.html?pagewanted=all)

Levi, Primo. *The Drowned and the Saved.* Trans. by Raymond Rosenthal. New York: Vintage International, 1989.

Levitin, Daniel J. *The World in Six Songs: How the Musical Brain Created Human Nature.* Toronto: Viking Canada, 2008.

MacDonald, Michael. *Mystical Bedlam; Madness, Anxiety, and Healing in Seventeenth-Century England.* Cambridge, U.K.: Cambridge University Press, 1981.

Macdonald, Nancy. "What a Waste," *Maclean's*, November 16, 2009. (http://www2.macleans.ca/2009/11/09/what-a-waste/)
———. "Who Needs A Break?" *Maclean's*, July 6, 2009, pp. 60-62. http://www2.macleans.ca/2009/07/01/who-needs-a-break/

McKinnell, Julia. "Survival Tips for the Nursing Home," *Maclean's*, June 30, 2009, p. 55.

McNeil, Donald G., Jr. "Far More Chinese Have Mental Disorders than Previously Reported, Study Finds," *The New York Times*, June 16, 2009, p. D6. (http://www.nytimes.com/2009/06/16/health/16glob.html)

Mendleson, Rachel. "Suicide Spree Hits France Telecom," *Maclean's*, October 26, 2009, p. 45. (http://www2.macleans.ca/2009/10/22/suicide-spree-hits-france-telecom/)

Orwell, George. *Homage to Catalonia.* London, Martin Secker & Warburg Ltd., 1938.
———. "Why I Write," in Daniel J. Leab (ed.), *Such, Such Were the Joys*, introduction by Richard Rovere. New York: Harcourt, Brace and Company, 1953

Pollan, Michael. *The Omnivore's Dilemma: A Natural History of Four Meals.* New York: Penguin Books, 2006.

Potter, Mitch. "Pills and America's Pursuit of Happiness," *Toronto Star*, September 2, 2009. (www.thestar.com/news/world/article/689697)

Seligman, Martin E. P. *Helplessness: On Depression, Development, and Death.* San Francisco: W.H. Freeman & Company, 1975.

Sapolsky, Robert M. *Why Zebras Don't Get Ulcers: An Updated Guide to Stress, Stress Related Diseases and Coping,* Second Edition. New York: Henry Holt and Company, 1994.

Shenk, Joshua Wolf. *Lincoln's Melancholy: How Depression Challenged a President and Fueled His Greatness.* New York: Houghton Mifflin, 2005.

Shwartz, Mark. "Robert Sapolsky Discusses Physiological Effects of Stress," *Stanford Report,* March 7, 2007. (http://news-service.stanford.edu/news/2006/november8/stress-110806.html)

Solomon, Andrew. *The Noonday Demon: An Atlas of Depression.* New York: Scribner, 2001.

Styron, William. *Darkness Visible: A Memoir of Madness.* New York: Vintage Books, 1990.

Tolstoy, Leo. *Anna Karenina.* New York: Barnes & Noble Classics, 2003.

Turner, Erick H., et al. Selective Publication of Antidepressant Trials and Its Influence on Apparent Efficacy," *The New England Journal of Medicine,* Volume 368: 252-260, Number 3, January 17, 2008.

U.S. Secret Service and U.S. Department of Education. *The Final Report and Findings of the Safe School Initiative: Implications for the Prevention of School Attacks in the United States,* May 2002.

Watters, Ethan. "The Americanization of Mental Illness," *The New York Times Sunday Magazine,* January 10, 2010, pp 40-45.

Wolpert, Lewis. *Malignant Sadness: The Anatomy of Depression.* New York: The Free Press, 1999.

Woolf, Virginia. "A Sketch of the Past," from Jeanne Schulkind (ed.), *Moments of Being.* London, Hogarth Press, 1985.
———. *Mrs. Dalloway.* London: Collector's Library, 2003.

About the Author

Jan Wong is an international best-selling author and award-winning foreign correspondent. She is a graduate of McGill University, Beijing University and Columbia University's Graduate School of Journalism. The recipient of the George Polk Award and a National Newspaper Award, among other honors for her reporting, she has written for the Montreal *Gazette*, *The New York Times*, *The Boston Globe*, *The Wall Street Journal* and *The Globe and Mail*.

Wong is the author of four other books: *Red China Blues, My Long March from Mao to Now*; *Jan Wong's China, Reports from a Not-So-Foreign Correspondent*; *Lunch With Jan Wong, Sweet and Sour Celebrity Interviews*; and *Beijing Confidential, a Tale of Comrades Lost and Found*. "Chinese Shadows," an upcoming documentary based on *Beijing Confidential*, is a co-production between two UK companies, Tigerlily Films and Sneak Preview Films.

In 2010, Wong was Visiting Irving Chair in Journalism at St. Thomas University in Fredericton. She currently divides her time between Toronto, where she is a columnist for *Toronto Life* magazine, and Fredericton, where she is a journalism professor at St. Thomas University.